HUMAN MILK BANKING

Human Milk Banking

Editors

A. F. Williams, M.R.C.P.

*Department of Paediatrics
John Radcliffe Hospital
Headington, Oxford, England*

J. D. Baum, M.D., F.R.C.P.

*Department of Paediatrics
John Radcliffe Hospital
Headington, Oxford, England*

Nestlé Nutrition
Workshop Series
Volume 5

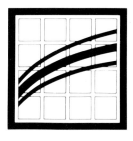

NESTLÉ NUTRITION, VEVEY

RAVEN PRESS ■ NEW YORK

Raven Press, 1140 Avenue of the Americas, new York, New York 10036

Made in the United States of America

Library of Congress Cataloging in Publication Data
Main entry under title:

Human milk banking.

    (Nestlé Nutrition workshop series; v. 5)
    Includes bibliographies and index.
    1. Milk, Human—Composition.   2. Infants (Newborn)—
Nutrition.   I. Williams, A. F. (Anthony Ffoulkes),
1951-   .   II. Baum, J. D.   III. Nestlé Nutrition S.A.
IV. Series.
QP246.H85   1984   613.2   84-17897
ISBN 0-88167-043-X (Raven Press)

    The material contained in this volume was submitted as previously unpublished material, except in the instances in which credit has been given to the source from which some of the illustrative material was derived.

    Great care has been taken to maintain the accuracy of the information contained in the volume. However, Nestlé Nutrition or Raven Press cannot be held responsible for errors or for any consequences arising from the use of the information contained herein.

Preface

The purpose in calling the meeting on which this volume is based was to consider the role of human milk and human milk fractions in the feeding of very-low-birth-weight infants. We sought to bring together investigators from many disciplines interested in this field to exchange information on the processing, biochemistry, and clinical applications of human milk fractions and fortified human milk.

It has long been recognized there are major problems in evaluating even the nutrition of term healthy infants. Although extremes of malnutrition are readily measurable, the only available short-term measures of nutrition for healthy infants are patterns of growth, complicated as they are by the enormous variability between babies from different families and environmental and racial backgrounds. Nevertheless, for the term infant at least, it is accepted that the appropriate food is the infant's own mother's fresh milk.

In the case of very-low-birth-weight preterm infants, the position is even more complex. Here, even growth is not a simple outcome measure given the profound influence of clinical factors other than nutrition, such as intracranial hemorrhage or respiratory failure, quite apart from the difficulties of providing appropriate extrauterine growth standards. These problems are further compounded in the long term by genetic and environmental influences. Although the identification of the proper food for such infants is fraught with difficulties, it remains likely that human milk and human milk products are the most appropriate food sources for such babies given the favorable amino acid composition of human milk proteins, the likely but unmeasured importance of the nonnutritional components of human milk, and the need to avoid nonhuman milk proteins with their potential for sensitization of the immature infant.

For these reasons it seemed worthwhile to provide a forum for investigators interested in the problems of human milk fractionation with a view to exchanging fundamental information on the processing and biological properties of human milk fractions and an evaluation of their use in clinical practice.

A. F. WILLIAMS
J. D. BAUM

Foreword

The advantages of breast milk for feeding normal term babies is beyond doubt. Breast milk expressed by mothers of low-birth-weight babies is also thought to offer the best nutrition for these infants, but there remains a good deal of controversy about feeding very-low-birth-weight (VLBW) infants with banked human milk. Thus, the energy, protein, and phosphorus requirements of VLBW infants may not be met adequately with the amount of banked human milk these infants can usually accept. Moreover, most hospital milk banks have problems in controlling the processing of human milk to maintain all the important qualities of human milk while minimizing the risk of transmitting infectious agents.

This book, the fifth in the *Nestlé Nutrition Workshop Series*, deals with some of the problems of feeding VLBW babies. It does not set out to give definitive answers, for, as one workshop participant remarked, we do not yet know all the questions. Nonetheless, there is much of interest in these contributions for all pediatricians, nutritionists, and others working to optimize the healthy survival of VLBW infants.

The Nestlé Nutrition Workshops concentrate on pediatric nutrition. Volumes already published in this series include *Maternal Nutrition in Pregnancy—Eating for Two?*, edited by J. Dobbing (Academic Press, 1981); *Acute Diarrhea: Its Nutritional Consequences in Children*, edited by J. A. Bellanti (Raven Press, 1983); *Nutritional Adaptation of the Gastrointestinal Tract of the Newborn*, edited by N. Kretchmer and A. Minkowski (Raven Press, 1983); *Chronic Diarrhea in Children*, edited by E. Lebenthal (Raven Press, 1984); *Iron Nutrition in Infancy and Childhood*, edited by A. Stekel (Raven Press, 1984). Forthcoming is *Nutritional Needs and Assessment for Normal Growth*, edited by M. Gracey and F. Falkner.

PIERRE R. GUESRY, M.D.
Vice President
Nestlé Products Technical
Assistance Co. Ltd.

Contents

ix

Contributors

S. Aubry
Lacterium de Paris
26 Boulevard Brune
Paris 75014, France

I. Axelsson
Department of Pediatrics
University of Lund
Malmö General Hospital
S-214 01 Malmö, Sweden

***V. Barrois-Larouze**
Lacterium de Paris
26 Boulevard Brune
75014 Paris, France

***J. D. Baum**
Department of Paediatrics
John Radcliffe Hospital
Oxford OX3 9DU, England

***Peter N. Campbell**
Courtauld Institute of
*   Biochemistry*
The Middlesex Hospital Medical
*   School*
Mortimer Street
London W1P 7PN, England

***Roger K. Craig**
Courtauld Institute of
*   Biochemistry*
The Middlesex Hospital Medical
*   School*
Mortimer Street
London W1P 7PN, England

Michael S. Davies
Courtauld Institute of
*   Biochemistry*
The Middlesex Hospital Medical
*   School*
Mortimer Street
London W1P 7PN, England

C. Dill
Department of Pediatrics
Baylor College of Medicine
1200 Moursund Avenue
Houston, Texas 77030, U.S.A.

J. Faber
Department of Pediatrics
Shaare Zedek Hospital
Jerusalem 91002, Israel

R. Fondén
Arla Research and Development
*   Department*
Stockholm, Sweden

***S. Freier**
Department of Pediatrics
Shaare Zedek Hospital
Jerusalem 91002, Israel

***C. Garza**
Department of Pediatrics
Baylor College of Medicine
1200 Moursund Avenue
Houston, Texas 77030, U.S.A.

---

*Conference participant.

xiii

*G. E. Gaull
*Institute of Basic Research in
  Mental Retardation
1050 Forest Hill Road
Staten Island, New York 10314
U.S.A.*

*F. A. Glover
*Process Technology Department
National Institute for Research in
  Dairying, Shinfield
Reading RG2 9AT, England*

A. S. Goldman
*Department of Pediatrics
Baylor College of Medicine
1200 Moursund Avenue
Houston, Texas, 77030, U.S.A.*

L. Grimonprez
*Laboratorire de Biochemie
Faculté de Pharmacie de
  Montpellier
Montpellier, France*

S. Hagelberg
*Department of Pediatrics
St. Göran's Children's Hospital
Box 12500
S-11281 Stockholm, Sweden*

Eveline D. Hall
*National Institute for Research in
  Dairying, Shinfield
Reading RG2 9AT, England*

Len Hall
*Courtauld Institute of
  Biochemistry
The Middlesex Hospital Medical
  School
Mortimer Street
London W1P 7PN, England*

*H. Hilpert
*Research Department
Nestlé Products Technical
  Assistance Co. Ltd.
CH-1814 La Tour de Peilz
Switzerland*

Manjit Hunjan
*National Institute for Research in
  Dairying
Hounslow TW3 4BW, England*

P. Hylmö
*Department of Pediatrics
University of Lund
Malmö General Hospital
S-214 01 Malmö, Sweden*

Charles E. Isaacs
*Institute of Basic Research in
  Mental Retardation
1050 Forest Hill Road
Staten Island, New York 10314
U.S.A.*

I. Jakobsson
*Department of Pediatrics
University of Lund
Malmö General Hospital
S-214 01 Malmö, Sweden*

Sylvie Jorieux
*Laboratoire de Chimie
  Biologique
Université des Sciences et
  Techniques de Lille I
59655 Villeneuve d'Ascq Cédex,
  France*

*Anne-Brit Kolstø Otnæss
*Vaccine Department
National Institute of Public
  Health
Oslo 1, Norway*

Leslie Krueger
*Institute of Basic Research in
    Mental Retardation
1050 Forest Hill Road
Staten Island, New York 10314
U.S.A.*

Astrid Lægreid
*Vaccine Department
National Institute of Public
    Health
Oslo 1, Norway*

*B. S. Lindblad
*Department of Pediatrics
St. Göran's Children's Hospital
Box 12500
S-11281 Stockholm, Sweden*

A. Lundsjö
*Department of Pediatrics
St. Göran's Children's Hospital
Box 12500
S-11281 Stockholm, Sweden*

*Richard L. J. Lyster
*National Institute for Research in
    Dairying, Shinfield
Reading RG2 9AT, England*

Joël Mazurier
*Laboratoire de Chimie
    Biologique
Université des Sciences et
    Techniques de Lille I
59655 Villeneuve d'Ascq Cédex,
    France*

Jean Montreuil
*Laboratoire de Chemie
    Biologique
Université des Sciences et
    Techniques de Lille I
59655 Villeneuve d'Ascq Cédex,
    France*

Jean Navarro
*Hôpital Bretonneau
Pavillon Legroux
75018 Paris, France*

B. L. Nichols
*Department of Pediatrics
Baylor College of Medicine
1200 Moursund Avenue
Houston, Texas 77030, U.S.A.*

Ivar Ørstavik
*Microbiological Laboratory
Ulleval Hospital
Oslo 1, Norway*

B. Persson
*Department of Pediatrics
St. Göran's Children's Hospital
Box 12500
S-11281 Stockholm, Sweden*

S. Polberger
*Department of Pediatrics
University of Lund
Malmö General Hospital
S-214 01, Malmö, Sweden*

Guy Putet
*University Hospital Edouard
    Herriot
Lyons, France*

*N. Räihä
*Department of Pediatrics
University of Lund
Malmö General Hospital
S-214 01 Malmö, Sweden*

*Bruno Reiter
*23 Brompton Court
Roy Park Avenue
Maidenhead
Berks SL6 8EA, England*

Jacques Rigo
Department of Neonatal
  Pediatrics
State University of Liège
Hôpital de Bavière
4020 Liège, Belgium

Charles Romond
Faculté de Pharmacie
Laboratoire de Microbiologie
59045 Lille Cédex, France

*R. J. Schanler
Department of Pediatrics
Baylor College of Medicine
1200 Moursund Avenue
Houston, Texas 77030, U.S.A.

*Jacques Senterre
Department of Neonatal
  Pediatrics
State University of Liège
Hôpital de Bavière
B-4020 Liège, Belgium

*Geneviève Spik
Laboratoire de Chimie
  Biologique
Université des Sciences et
  Techniques de Lille I
59655 Villeneuve d'Ascq Cédex,
  France

Harris H. Tallan
Institute of Basic Research in
  Mental Retardation
1050 Forest Hill Road
Staten Island, New York 10314,
  U.S.A.

Karin Trollerud
Vaccine Department
National Institute of Public
  Health
Oslo 1, Norway

Marcel Voyer
Institut de Puériculture de Paris
Paris, France

*A. F. Williams
Department of Paediatrics
John Radcliffe Hospital
Oxford OX3 9DU, England

Charles E. Wright
Institute of Basic Research in
  Mental Retardation
1050 Forest Hill Road
Staten Island, New York 10314,
  U.S.A.

Invited Attendees

K. Amatayakul/*Chiangmai,*
  Thailand
S. Calvert/*Oxford, England*
P. Cheeseman/*London, England*
P. Chowanich/*Chiangmai,*
  Thailand
E. DeMaeyer/*Geneva,*
  Switzerland

J. Dobbing/*Manchester, England*
J. A. Dodge/*Cardiff, Wales*
S. R. Fine/*London, England*
C. Fisher/*Oxford, England*
S. Flache/*Zurich, Switzerland*
S. Forsey/*Windsor, England*
V. Greasley/*Oxford, England*

J. Harrington/*Windsor, England*
D. Harris/*Oxford, England*
D. Hull/*Nottingham, England*
P. Jenkins/*Oxford, England*
T. Lesoli/*Oxford, England*
R. Lindemann/*Oslo, Norway*
A. Lucas/*Cambridge, England*
R. Preston/*Oxford, England*
J. D. Priddle/*Oxford, England*
S. Silpisornkosol/*Chiangmai, Thailand*

W. A. Silverman/*Greenbrae, California, U.S.A.*
G. Soltesz/*Oxford, England*
T. E. T. Stacey/*Middlesex, England*
B. Wharton/*Birmingham, England*
A. R. Wilkinson/*Oxford, England*
M. Woolridge/*Oxford, England*

Nestlé Participants

S. R. Allen
Nestlé Products Technical Assistance Co. Ltd. La Tour de Peilz, Switzerland

Pierre R. Guesry
Vice President Nestlé Products Technical Assistance Co. Ltd. La Tour de Peilz, Switzerland

H. Hilpert
Research Department Nestlé Products Technical Assistance Co. Ltd. La Tour de Peilz, Switzerland

G. A. Raffe
The Nestlé Co. Ltd. Croydon, England

HUMAN MILK BANKING

Human Milk Banking, edited by
A. F. Williams and J. D. Baum.
Nestlé Nutrition, Vevey/Raven Press,
New York © 1984.

Principles of Ultrafiltration and the Concentration and Fractionation of Cow's Milk

F. A. Glover

Process Technology Department, National Institute for Research in Dairying, Shinfield, Reading RG2 9AT, England

The principle of ultrafiltration (UF) is filtration of solutions or suspensions under pressure through a semipermeable membrane. The membrane has pores that allow the solvent and small molecules to pass through and the larger molecules to be retained. Ultrafiltration may therefore be considered as both a concentration and a fractionation process according to the particular components of interest.

Ultrafiltration is often associated with reverse osmosis (RO), sometimes called hyperfiltration, and UF and RO are known as membrane processes. The association exists because both are pressure-driven processes, the apparatus and plants for each look very similar, and originally cellulose acetate was the base material of the membranes for both processes. But RO membranes do not have pores and are permeable only to water, so that RO is purely a concentration process. The principle of RO is quite different from that of UF. Water passes through an RO membrane by a solution/diffusion process and is opposed by the osmotic pressure of the solution being concentrated so that far higher pressures are used for RO than for UF.

Ultrafiltration has been used for a long time in the laboratory. For example, a most readable review of UF on this scale was

1

produced by Ferry in 1936 (1). More recently Glover et al. (2) have reviewed membrane processing with particular reference to milk and whey. The current interest in membrane processing arose from the discovery (3) just before 1960 of the technique of making cellulose acetate membranes on a large scale for commercial use. Reverse osmosis received the initial impetus from the American desalination program. This was then followed by developments in UF when it was realized that UF has a much wider application and that better membranes could be made from other materials.

THE FILTER RANGE

Ultrafiltration serves to concentrate molecules in the size range 1 μm down to 10^{-3} μm, filtering out molecules below this level. This is the range of colloidal particles and macromolecules, including, for example, the casein micelle with a diameter of 10^{-1} μm. The filter range is shown in Fig. 1 together with the sizes of the components of milk. This puts UF into perspective with other types of filtration.

THE ULTRAFILTRATION PROCESS

The simplest form of UF in the laboratory employs a sheet of membrane supported on a grid near the bottom of a closed beaker in which pressure can be maintained in the region of 200 to 500

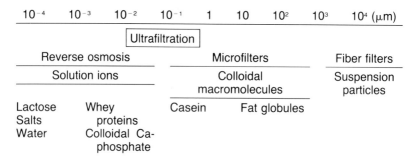

FIG. 1.   The filter range.

kPa (2–5 bar). A magnetic stirrer must be operated in the solution, and the arrangement is known as the stirred cell. A more sophisticated laboratory approach uses membranes in tubular or plate-and-frame assemblies and a peristaltic pump to provide a flow of the feed over the membrane. On the industrial scale, the same principle is scaled up to various levels of engineering sophistication incorporating pressure, flow, and temperature monitoring and automatic control. Plants are rated in terms of their membrane areas, which can be 100s or 1,000s of square meters.

The performance of the membrane is described by its retention of the large molecules and its rate of filtration, the permeate flux. If C_f is the concentration of a component of the feed, and C_p is the concentration of that component in the permeate, then retention R is given by

$$R = [(C_f - C_p)/C_f] \times 100$$

In the ideal ultrafiltration of milk, R is 100% for casein and 0% for lactose.

Permeate flux is measured in liters per hour per square meter of membrane and quoted under standard conditions of operating pressure and temperature. Fluxes occur in the region of 150 liters m^{-2} hr^{-1} at 25°C for water, and 50 liters m^{-2} hr^{-1} at 50°C for milk at normal ($\times 1$) concentration.

The most important aspects of an understanding of the principle of UF are the mass transfer through the membrane and the consequences of that transfer on the feed side of the membrane, where filtration is to proceed. Consider Fig. 2, representing a feed (milk) entering a tubular membrane from the left, having a permeate containing lactose, salts, and water removed by ultrafiltration and leaving on the right a product concentrated in fat and protein. The properties of the membrane that will affect its permeability are its pore size, its thickness, and its hydrophilic nature. The properties of the permeate that will affect its rate of flow will be the molecular sizes and shapes of its components, its viscosity, and its temperature, insofar as temperature will affect viscosity. Since the process is driven by pressure, the flux will be directly proportional to the

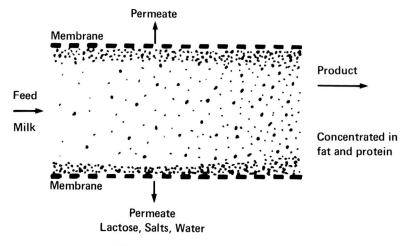

FIG. 2.   Concentration polarization.

pressure difference across the membrane, but some of the applied pressure will be dissipated by the opposing viscous forces as the feed flows along the membrane tube. Hence, the pressure available for ultrafiltration will decrease as the feed moves along the tube.

At the membrane surface (the site of filtration), the retained molecules will collect and be concentrated as the permeate is extracted. Unless they are dispersed, they will hinder further filtration, and the permeate flux will fall. To ensure that the process continues, high rates of shear or large degrees of turbulence must be employed to move the solids away from the membrane and assist them to diffuse back into the main stream of the flow. Nevertheless, by the nature of the process, there will always be a higher concentration of solids near the membrane than in the main body of the feed. This increase of concentration in the direction towards the membrane is termed concentration polarization. Concentration polarization can never be eliminated; it can only be minimized. Equilibrium is set up between the rate at which solids are left at the membrane by the removal of permeate and the rate of their assisted diffusion back into the main flow of the feed. The level of concentration polarization will increase as the concentration factor of the feed increases; hence, the permeate flux declines as concentration proceeds. In Fig. 2, concentration is proceeding as the feed moves to the right; hence, concentration polarization is more serious the longer the membrane tube. The polarized layer forms within seconds of the start of filtration, causing a rapid initial decline in flux. Flux can be increased by higher flow rates of the feed, but a compromise with energy expended in pumping must be accepted. In practice, flow velocities over the membrane in the region of 5 m/sec are used.

As concentration polarization increases, solids are deposited on the surface of the membrane and in the pores. To some extent deposition occurs after any ultrafiltration of milk, as demonstrated by measuring a pure water flux immediately afterwards and finding that it is considerably reduced from the level obtainable from a cleaned membrane. This deposit acts as a secondary membrane, greatly influencing the rate of filtration. Table 1 gives examples of thicknesses of deposits recovered from membranes that have ultrafiltered aqueous protein solutions at the concentrations listed.

Since the fluxes obtained from skimmed milk are only a little higher than those from whole milk, it is evident that fat is not the main hindrance to the process. Deposits consist mainly of protein: in the case of cow's milk, β-lactoglobulin is responsible for the greatest decline in flux because of its ability to form layers of material (5).

TABLE 1. *Deposits on the membrane during UF of aqueous protein solution*[a]

Protein (%)	Deposit thickness (μm)
1	0.1–0.3
4	0.7–2
12.8	6–12

[a]From ref. 4.

Following this description of the process, the factors governing the rate of ultrafiltration may be appreciated in summary:

1. area of membrane;
2. length of membrane;
3. pressure difference across the membrane;
4. rate of shear at the membrane surface or degree of turbulence in the flow stream;
5. concentration of the feed;
6. viscosity of the concentrate;
7. viscosity of the permeate;
8. hydrodynamic resistance of the membrane; and
9. hydrodynamic resistance of the deposited layer.

DIAFILTRATION

Since the small molecules and water pass through the membrane together, the concentrations of these components in the water phase in both the concentrate and the permeate will be the same. Thus, in the ultrafiltration of milk in which the concentration of lactose is initially about 4.8%, provided the retention of lactose during ultrafiltration is zero, the concentration of lactose in the permeate will also be about 4.8%, since both milk and permeate are approximately dilute aqueous solutions. If milk is diluted with water and ultrafiltration is continued, lactose will be removed with the permeate, producing a low-lactose milk. At the same time, the salts content will be similarly reduced. This combined process of dilution and ultrafiltration to wash out the permeating components is known as diafiltration. The usual method is to add water at the same rate as the permeate is being removed. Levels of the retained components may be adjusted as required by the appropriate amount of ultrafiltration.

If milk is taken as an example, a low-lactose milk of required composition may be prepared as follows (6): If

m_w Mass of water in the milk before diafiltration
l_1 Mass of lactose in the milk before diafiltration
l_2 Mass of lactose required in the low-lactose milk
R Retention coefficient of lactose (which in practice is not zero)
V Volume of water to be added

then
$$V = \frac{m_w}{1 - R} \cdot \ln \frac{l_1}{l_2}$$

MEMBRANE COMPOSITION AND STRUCTURE

The first membranes were made of cellulose acetate. The cellulose molecule consists of two glucose units, each with three hydroxyl groups. Replacement of an average of 2.5 of these hydroxyl groups by acetyl groups produces the base for an ultrafiltration membrane. The breakthrough in membrane technology came with the discovery that it was possible to make a membrane with a very thin surface layer—the layer that is effectively the filter—supported on a much thicker and much more porous sublayer, which gives strength to the whole structure. These are the so-called asymmetric membranes now in general use. The thickness of the whole membrane is of the order of 100 μm, most of which is the sponge-like sublayer supporting the filtering layer, which is ~0.25 μm thick. This structure is illustrated in Fig. 3.

The early membranes were made by dissolving cellulose acetate in acetone and adding a small quantity of magnesium perchlorate to serve as a swelling agent. This formed a gel from which the perchlorate could be leached out to leave a system of interconnecting pores. Heating the surface of this gel produced the tight skin, the thin ultrafiltration layer. Different porosities could be made by varying the time/temperature relationship of the heat treatment. The permeability of the layer is chosen as a compromise between a desirable permeate flux and a permissible loss of components from the concentrate.

Cellulose acetate as a material for membranes has some limitations, particularly for use on biological systems. Since it is an ester

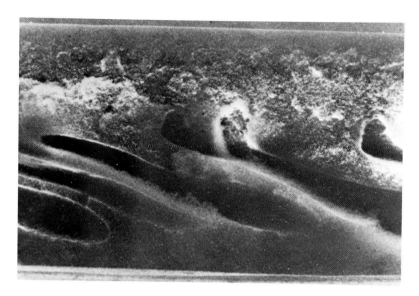

FIG. 3. Structure of UF membrane. Electron micrograph of cross section of polysulfone UF membrane, ×500, showing sponge-like underlayer and upper layer of much greater density. (From ref. 7.)

and a polysaccharide, it is subject to hydrolysis, which limits its use to a pH range of 3 to 7 and an upper temperature limit of 35°C. It can also be affected by alcohols, some organic acids, and some bacteria. All of these impose limitations on the use and cleaning and sterilization of cellulose acetate membranes.

For these reasons they have now been superseded, first by polyamide and later by polysulfone membranes. The polysulfones are much more tolerant to temperature and pH, withstanding temperatures up to 80°C and pH values from 2 to 12. They also have better resistance to chlorine, compaction under pressure, and electrochemical action. The polysulfone membranes are now, in turn, being challenged by inorganic membranes of zirconium oxide made integral with their graphite supports. These are unaffected by temperatures up to 400°C, by pH values over the whole range 0 to 14, and by pressures up to 4 MPa (40 bar) and have great mechanical strength.

MEMBRANE CUT-OFF LEVELS

Membranes are made with stated molecular weight cut-off levels covering a very wide range, from 1,000 to 100,000. However, such specifications must be regarded as a guide rather than an expectation of performance. The size and shape of molecules more than their weight will govern their passage through a membrane, and the size distribution of pores in the membrane is more likely to be diffuse than sharp. Furthermore, in practice, deposits on the membrane will greatly modify the permeability of the system. Membranes used in milk processing have cut-off levels in the 5,000 to 20,000 molecular weight region.

MEMBRANE GEOMETRY

Membranes may be flat or tubular. They are attached to a supporting porous backing, which in turn is further supported by an outer perforated plate or tube. The most characteristic dimension of an assembly is the width of the flow channel between adjacent membranes, i.e., the space between the flat sheets or the internal diameter of the tubular forms. Flow channels between flat sheets are 0.5 mm to 2.5 mm wide; tube diameters range from 6 mm to 25 mm. Variations on these two configurations exist in flat membranes rolled into spirals and in tubular forms being reduced to 1 to 2 mm internal diameter, then known as hollow fibers.

The unit in membrane assemblies is called the module. This is either a pile of plates, a bundle of fibers or tubes, or a spirally wound assembly. Sizes of modules are quoted in areas of membrane that range from a few hundredths of a square meter for the laboratory to about 50 m^2 per module on the industrial scale.

ULTRAFILTRATION PLANT AND OPERATION

Apart from the membrane module assembly, the components of an ultrafiltration plant are normal centrifugal pumps, valves, pressure gauges, heat exchangers, all constructed in stainless steel to required hygienic standards if milk or whey is to be processed. Entrance and exit pressures for the membrane section are usually about 5 bar and 2 bar; flow rates are in the region of 500 liters min^{-1}; and the operating temperature is 50°C, safely below the temperature at which the whey proteins start to denature and away from the temperature most favorable to bacterial growth at 37°C. To reach any appreciable concentration, the milk must pass over the membrane many times. Operation can be either in a batch system, whereby after each pass the milk is returned to the starting tank, or in a continuous system, in which the milk is circulated over the membrane in a closed loop. A little of the concentrate is bled off continuously, and more feed is introduced at the entrance of the loop to keep the volume constant. In this latter method, the average retention time of the milk in the plant is reduced to a few minutes, which restrains bacterial growth. When this system is used industrially, during each 24-hr period the plant is run for 20 hr and is cleaned for 4 hr. Cleaning is with detergent to remove the fat, sodium hypochlorite or enzyme to break down the protein, and nitric acid to remove the minerals. Under these conditions, the life of a membrane is guaranteed for 1 year.

MILK PROPERTIES RELEVANT TO ULTRAFILTRATION

The composition of cow's milk is given in Table 2, and the corresponding molecular sizes are shown in Table 3. It can be seen from Tables 2 and 3 how appropriate ultrafiltration is for the separation of proteins from the lactose and salts in milk. Between α-

TABLE 2. *Composition of cow's milk*

Component	Concentration (%)	Chemical nature	Physical state
Fat	3.8	Triglycerides	Emulsion
Protein	3.2	Caseins; whey proteins	Colloidal solution
Lactose	4.8		Solution
Minerals	0.7	Calcium phosphate	Bound and free
		Citrates	Solution
		Na and K chlorides	Solution

TABLE 3. *Molecular sizes of milk components[a]*

Component	Molecular weight	Diameter (nm)
Fat globule	—	4,000
Casein micelle	10^7-10^9	100
Blood serum albumin	69,000	5
β-Lactoglobulin	36,000	4
α-Lactalbumin	14,500	3
Lactose	342	0.8
Ca^{2+}	40	0.4
Cl^-	35	0.4
Water	18	0.3

[a]From ref. 8.

lactalbumin and lactose there is a very convenient large size interval at a level to suit the pore size of easily made UF membranes. The tables also illustrate that for filtration purposes it is much more realistic to think in terms of molecular dimensions than molecular weights, which could give misleading impressions of size.

Milk is by no means a commodity of constant composition. It varies with

individuality of the cow,
breed,
feed,
age of the cow,
stage of lactation,
season, and
milking procedure.

However, on the industrial scale, large quantities of milk are bulked together, smoothing out these variations.

Viscosity is the most important physical property of milk relevant to ultrafiltration. Casein makes the largest single contribution to the viscosity of milk, rather more than the fat and considerably more than the whey proteins, the lactose, and the salts. Since casein plays such a major role, factors affecting the stability of casein, such as acidity, salt balance, and heat treatment, will all influence viscosity. As concentration by ultrafiltration proceeds, the viscosity of milk increases markedly. For example, the viscosity of skimmed milk, which is ~1.5 cP at 25°C at its normal solids concentration of 8.5%, increases sevenfold as ultrafiltration increases the solids content to 30%.

THE RATE OF ULTRAFILTRATION OF MILK

If whole milk is concentrated by ultrafiltration as a batch process, the permeate flux declines with the increase in concentration, as in Fig. 4. The concentration factor is the ratio in which the starting volume of the milk is reduced, which will also be the factor by which the concentrations of the fat and protein are increased if the retentions of these components are 100%, as is usually the case.

It will be seen that the practical limit of concentration is about four- to fivefold. Taking the composition of the starting milk from Table 2, the approximate composition of the concentrate is given in Table 4. In practice, it is found that the retention of lactose may be up to 10%.

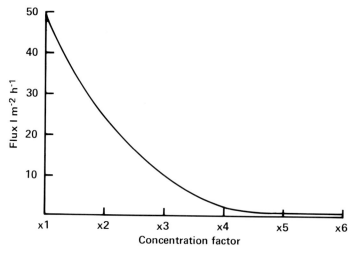

FIG. 4. Ultrafiltration of milk. Decline of flux as concentration increases.

TABLE 4. *Composition of the concentrate*

Component	Amount[a] (%)
Fat	15.2
Protein	12.8
Lactose	3.7
Minerals	0.6
Water	67.8

[a]Calculated on the basis of zero lactose retention.

If ultrafiltration is carried out on a feed and bleed principle, the average concentration factor in the membrane loop will be close to the final level. Hence, the flux curve will decline initially as in Fig. 4 and then continue horizontally near the required concentration for the main processing time.

For the concentration of skimmed milk, the flux curve will be a few, ($\simeq$5) liters per square meter per hour above that for whole milk. Since the rate of filtration is controlled by the protein content of the feed, the flux from whey will be still higher and decline less rapidly with increase in concentration factor than the flux from skimmed milk. However, at comparable protein levels in whole milk, skimmed milk, and whey, the permeate fluxes are similar. The protein concentration in a 25-fold whey concentrate is about the same as in a fourfold milk concentrate. It is therefore possible to concentrate whey up to 20- to 30-fold.

APPLICATIONS OF ULTRAFILTRATION IN DAIRYING

The main application is for the manufacture of soft cheese, to incorporate the whey proteins and so increase the yield of cheese (9).

Whey is the liquid drained from cheese curd during cheesemaking. From 10 kg of milk, the yield of hard cheese is approximately 1 kg and 9 kg of whey is discharged, taking with it 50% of the solids in the original milk. The composition of rennet whey from cheddar cheesemaking is given in Table 5. Milk ultrafiltrate consists of water, lactose, and salts; whey consists of water, protein, lactose, and salts. If for making cheese, milk is first concentrated by UF to a point at which there will be no further liquid to drain after the coagulation stage, i.e., no whey, the whey proteins will be retained in the cheese. This process is now established in industry with the advantage of an improved yield of cheese of about 15%. It is applicable only to the manufacture of soft cheeses, which have high water contents (in excess of 60%) that can be reached in the ultrafiltration stage. Milk is first concentrated up to fivefold, forming a "precheese." Starter and rennet are added, and the precheese is put directly into molds where coagulation takes place. Several types of soft cheese are now being made in this way, the largest production being in feta cheese, for which an increased yield of 21% above yields by traditional methods is claimed.

The same technique cannot be applied directly to the making of hard cheese, since milk cannot be concentrated to the level of the total solids in hard cheese, $\simeq 62\%$. Development is in progress using a combination of UF and evaporation for making the harder cheeses (10).

TABLE 5. *Composition of rennet whey*

Component	Amount (%)
Lactose	4.9
Protein	0.5
Nonprotein nitrogen	0.4
Fat	0.3
Ash	0.6
Lactic acid	0.2
Water	93
Whey proteins	
β-Lactoglobulin	
α-Lactalbumin	
Blood serum albumin	
Immunoglobulins	
Lactoferrin	

Ultrafiltration of whey is practiced primarily to combat the problem of disposal of the large volumes of a liquid with very high biological oxygen demand (BOD) values and, secondly, to make better use of valuable nutrients than has been done hitherto. By a combination of UF to concentrate the protein, diafiltration to remove the lactose, and, finally, drying, a whey protein concentrate is being produced. It contains approximately 75% protein in dry matter and is used in the meat and bakery industries where its good functional properties make it an excellent substitute for egg white.

Extraction of the protein from whey does not solve the pollution problem, since the BOD resides in the permeate, which is mainly a lactose solution. Lactose is not of great nutritional value, but if it is hydrolyzed into its two component monosaccharides, glucose and galactose, a sweet syrup is produced. This can be done with mineral acids, ion-exchange resins, or by enzyme action. A process has been developed in which the permeate is passed through a column of silica beads holding the enzyme β-galactosidase (11). Over 90% of the lactose is hydrolyzed, and the product is used in the bakery, confectionery, and ice cream trades.

Alternatively, the lactose in the permeate can be fermented to produce alcohol. The process is already in commercial operation (12).

RECENT DEVELOPMENTS IN ULTRAFILTRATION

With improvements in membrane technology, the pore size distribution is becoming better defined. As an extension of the above separation of whole protein, there is now promise of fractionating individual whey proteins (13). There is a proposal for using ultrafiltration to produce an α-lactalbumin-enriched fraction from whey. Such a product would be of great interest in the medical field in the humanizing of cows' milk, since α-lactalbumin is the main protein in human milk. If whey is ultrafiltered over a membrane having a cut-off level of 20,000 molecular weight, the β-lactoglobulin will be retained, and the α-lactalbumin will pass into the permeate. A second stage of ultrafiltration using a membrane with a 2,000 molecular weight cut-off for this permeate will retain and concentrate the α-lactalbumin.

The enzymatic membrane reactor technique is suggesting new uses. If an enzyme reaction is conducted in a container lined with an appropriate UF membrane, the breakdown products of the action will be passed through the membrane and can be collected, and the enzyme can be retained for further use. In this way, the initial steps of human digestion can be carried out *in vitro*, enabling predigested proteins to be collected in the permeate (13). Such a product would be helpful to those suffering digestive disorders, and indeed it is known that a demand for predigested proteins exists.

Ultrafiltration on a laboratory or industrial scale offers the possibility of selectively concentrating the components of cow's milk. This is an important development for the bovine dairy industry and provides a valuable model for those interested in the fractionation of milk.

REFERENCES

1. Ferry JD. Chem Rev 1936;18:373–455.
2. Glover FA, Skudder PJ, Stothart PH, Evans EW. J Dairy Res 1978;45:291–318.
3. Loeb S, Sourirajan S. University of California Los Angeles Department of Engineering Report 60–60. Los Angeles: University of California Press, 1960.
4. Kessler HG. In: Food engineering and dairy technology. Freising, FRG: Verlag A. Kessler, 1981:94.
5. Lee DN, Miranda MG, Merson RL. J Food Technol 1975;10:139–46.
6. Peri C, Pompei C, Rossi F. J Food Sci 1973;38:135–40.
7. Madsen RF. Hyperfiltration and ultrafiltration in plate and frame systems. Amsterdam: Elsevier, 1977:235.
8. Kessler HG. Food engineering and dairy technology. Freising, FRG: Verlag A. Kessler, 1981:84.
9. Maubois JL, Mocquot GP, Vassal LJ. Offenlegungschrift 2035 534. Bonn: German Patent Office, 1971, FRG.
10. Sutherland BJ, Jameson GW. Aust J Dairy Technol 1981;36:136–43.
11. Dicker R. Dairy Ind Int 1982;47(4):19–21.
12. Barry JA. Dairy Ind Int 1982;47(10):19–22.
13. Roger L. Contribution à la recherche d'une meilleure utilisation en alimentation humaine des composants glucidiques et protéiques du lactoserum grâce à l'emploi des techniques à membrane [Thesis]. Rennes, France: University of Rennes, 1979.

Human Milk Banking, edited by
A. F. Williams and J. D. Baum.
Nestlé Nutrition, Vevey/Raven Press,
New York © 1984.

Preparation of a Milk Immunoglobulin Concentrate from Cow's Milk

H. Hilpert

Research Department, Nestlé Products Technical Assistance Co. Ltd.,
CH-1814 La Tour de Peilz, Switzerland

There cannot be any serious doubt about the superiority of breast milk in the nutrition of the healthy term infant (1–3). However, it is frequently impossible for preterm infants and very-low-birth-weight infants to be nourished with their own mothers' milk. They must therefore depend on banked human milk if they are to profit from the nutritional and immunological advantages of human milk.

The relatively high protein and energy requirements of the low-birth-weight preterm infant suggest that pooled human milk may have nutritional inadequacies (4,5). The concept of a human milk formula was proposed in order to meet these nutritional requirements (6–10).

To maximize the advantage of protein enrichment of human milk, care should be taken to insure that the human milk protein isolate has fully preserved immunobiological properties. From our work on the immunobiological modification of cow's milk infant formulas, we have gathered some experience in the isolation of a "milk immunoglobulin concentrate" (MIC) from cow's milk (11,12). This chapter describes the isolation procedure employed in the hope that it will be of use to those who work on adapting human milk.

17

THE RATIONALE FOR MILK
IMMUNOGLOBULIN CONCENTRATE

Modern infant milk formulas attempt to provide nutritional equivalence to human milk, but even the most sophisticated products are devoid of any protective immune factors. We consider this to be a serious deficiency, especially when a formula is used to feed high-risk infants such as the very-low-birth-weight infant, who is prone to antibiotic-resistant nosocomial infections.

Immunoglobulins (Ig) are thought to play an important role among the protective immune factors in human milk. We have therefore investigated the possibility that these human milk immunoglobulins can be replaced by bovine milk immunoglobulins when babies are formula fed.

To reach this goal, a number of preliminary steps were essential:

1. Defining the specificity of bovine milk Ig.
2. Measuring the resistance of bovine milk Ig to proteolytic digestion.
3. Measuring the efficacy of bovine milk Ig in impeding the pathological mechanisms of common neonatal bacterial pathogens.
4. Demonstrating the clinical efficiency of bovine-Ig-enriched milk formulas.
5. Developing a technological treatment of the antibody-containing milk that insures bacteriological safety of the product while conserving its immunobiological activity. It is the last point that will be described in most detail in this present chapter.

Bovine milk immunoglobulins are part of the whey protein fraction. In order to avoid unnecessary losses of product and activity, we have not set out to isolate a pure immunoglobulin fraction but rather to separate the total whey proteins including the immunoglobulins, serum albumin, α-lactalbumin, β-lactoglobulin, and some minor proteins including bovine milk lactoferrin. The term MIC is justified when it is prepared from milk collected during the first 30 days of lactation, thus including colostral milk (see Fig. 1). This

Distribution of constituents in milk of first 30 days of lactation:

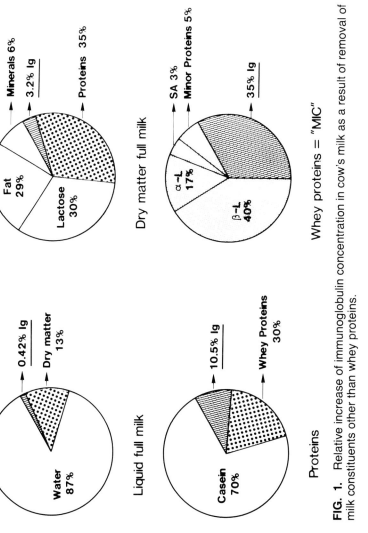

Liquid full milk

Proteins

Whey proteins = "MIC"

FIG. 1. Relative increase of immunoglobulin concentration in cow's milk as a result of removal of milk constituents other than whey proteins.

milk contains on an average 0.42% total Ig. Removal of water results in a dry matter containing 3.2% Ig. Elimination of lactose, fat, and minerals gives a protein fraction with 10.5% Ig. The separation of casein finally results in a whey protein fraction containing 35% Ig.

THE TECHNOLOGY OF MIC PREPARATION

Figure 2 shows the general flow sheet for MIC preparation.

Untreated raw milk—especially colostral milk—sometimes contains blood and other cellular material. In order to remove erythrocytes, other cells, and coarse impurities, the cold milk ($+8°C$ to $+12°C$) is centrifuged in a regular milk separator. Separation into skim milk and fat is achieved by running the milk through the same centrifuge after heating the milk to $+40°C$.

In order to accumulate the necessary quantities of milk for batch handling, the skim milk is kept frozen at $-25°C$. We have not observed any loss of antibody activity using this method of storage.

In order to inactivate any contaminating viruses, the thawed skimmed milk is heated to $+56°C$ in a plate heat exchanger. The milk is held at this temperature for 30 min in a jacketed vat equipped with a stirrer before cooling to $+37°C$.

At $+37°C$, the milk casein is precipitated by acidification to pH 4.5 or coagulated by renneting. To obtain a good contraction of the curd, the coagulated milk is heated once more to $+56°C$ for 10 min.

A first separation of lactoserum from precipitated casein is done by simple decantation followed by two washings of the casein slurry with demineralized water. By centrifugation in a clarifier centrifuge, the casein is separated from the last washing. The original lactoserum and the casein washings, which are kept separately, are finally cleared of all fine particles by successive passage through the same centrifuge followed by filtration through a depth filter of the Seitz or Filtrox type. This final clarification is an essential step in order to avoid obstruction problems in the ultrafiltration procedure that follows.

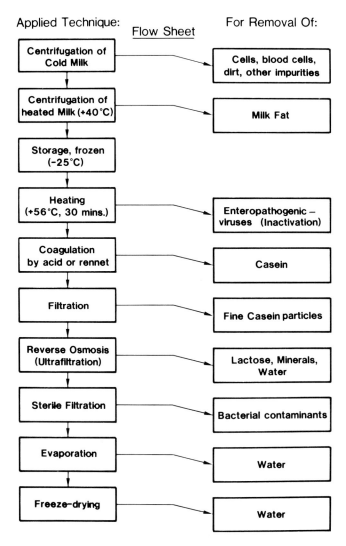

FIG. 2. General flow sheet showing the applied techniques for the preparation of milk immunoglobulin concentrate from cow's milk.

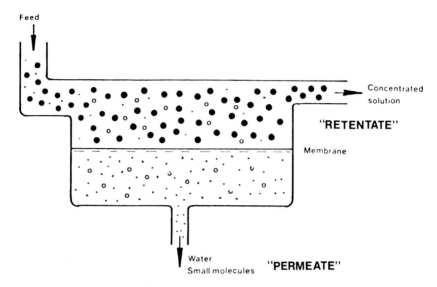

FIG. 3. Principle of ultrafiltration.

Ultrafiltration (principle described in Fig. 3) is carried out in a membrane-type installation in order to remove the bulk of lactose and mineral salts. By the application of positive pressure on a constantly circulating solution, water and small-molecular-weight substances are forced to penetrate the membrane and are removed with the permeate. High-molecular-weight material cannot pass through the membrane and is preserved in the retentate. This separation according to molecular size depends, of course, on the type of membrane employed. We use a DDS (Danish Sugar Corporation) unit that is equipped with the membrane type GR 81 P, whose properties together with those of other possible membrane types are given in Table 1.

Ultrafiltration is divided into 3 steps:

1. preconcentration;
2. diafiltration; and
3. final concentration.

In the preconcentration step, the original lactoserum is concentrated three- to fourfold. In the diafiltration step, the volume of the

TABLE 1. *Properties of DDS ultrafiltration membranes*[a]

Membrane type	Water capacity (liters/ m²/hr)	Lactose permeability (%)	Approx. cut-off value MW	Recommended operation range		
				pH	°C	MPa
500	300	100	65,000	2–8	0–50	0–0.5
600	150	98	20,000	2–8	0–50	0–1
800	80	95	6,000	2–8	0–50	0–2
GR61P	350	98	20,000	0–14	0–80	0–1.5
GR81P	100	95	6,000	0–14	0–80	0–1.5
FS60PP	300	100	30,000	0–13	0–80	0–1
GR60P	350	98	25,000	1–13	0–80	0–1

[a]Data measured after 1 hr of operation at 0.5 MPa (72.5 psi), +20°C. (From DDS membrane data sheet, DDS-Nakskov, Denmark.)

retentate is kept constant by the successive addition of the two casein washings. The final concentration reduces the concentrate volume another twofold. This procedure is summarized in Fig. 4.

The resulting whey protein solution with 10% dry matter, 7 to 8% total protein, and 2 to 3% Ig is now submitted to sterile filtration. In order to avoid premature clogging of the sterile filter, careful prefiltration of the protein solution is extremely important. Seitz or Filtrox depth filter plates, type Supra EK, are used for prefiltration. Sterile filtration is accomplished by a combination of Seitz or Filtrox depth filter plates, type EKS, and a Millipore® membrane filter with 0.45-μm pore size.

In order to reduce the volume for the final step of drying by lyophilization, the sterile whey protein solution undergoes evaporation of water at low temperature and reduced pressure in a thin-film evaporator. The material is exposed to a maximum temperature of +40°C. Our evaporation installation is equipped to run under sterile conditions.

The concentrated whey protein solution with about 20% dry matter, 14 to 16% total protein, and 4 to 6% Ig is finally dried by freeze-drying under sterile conditions. We use a small production-sized freeze-dryer from Usifroid with a condenser capacity of 50 kg water. The composition of the resulting powder is shown in Table

Ultrafiltration of Lactoserum:

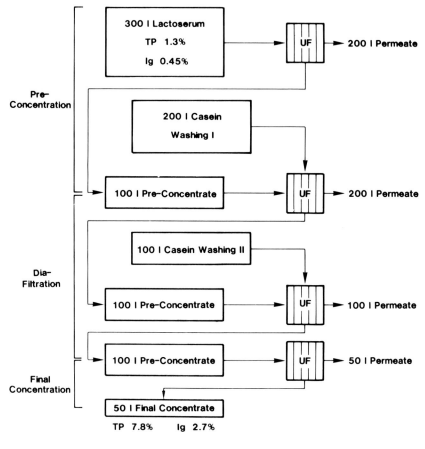

FIG. 4. Ultrafiltration of 300 liters of lactoserum with indication of retentate and permeate volumes in the course of preconcentration, diafiltration, and final concentration.

TABLE 2. *Average composition of an MIC isolated from cow's milk from the first 30 days of lactation*

Component	Amount (%)
Proteins	75 ± 5
Immunoglobulins	40 ± 5
IgG$_1$	75
IgG$_2$	3
IgA	17
IgM	6
α-Lactalbumin	15 ± 5
β-Lactoglobulin	35 ± 5
Serum albumin	3 ± 2
Minor proteins	5 ± 2
Residual humidity	4 ± 0.5
Residual lactose	10 ± 2
Residual mineral salts	5 ± 2
Nonprotein nitrogen compounds	5 ± 2

2. It can easily be mixed with milk powder and is perfectly soluble in water or liquid milk.

DISCUSSION

None of the applied techniques is new, but their combination, as described here, is of relevance to the preparation of a human milk protein isolate. A problem that will arise concerns the volume of milk to be treated. We work with volumes varying between 200 and 500 liters of milk from immunized cows, but smaller quantities of milk will be available in the case of human milk. This does not affect the fundamental approach described here but will affect the type of equipment used. Therefore, Table 3 not only shows the description of the installation as it is used in our work but also proposes alternatives that might be useful for work with smaller milk volumes. These indications do not claim to represent the best solution. That could only be established after careful investigations by milk engineering specialists.

TABLE 3. *Preparation of MIC from cow's milk: technical equipment and possible alternatives for smaller milk volumes*

Procedure	Equipment used for 200–500 kg full cow's milk	Equipment proposed for 20–50 kg full human milk
Centrifugation for milk clarification and skimming	Diabolo milk separator, type AE-574 Throughput max., 500 liters/hr	Alfa Perfect milk separator type AE-31 Throughput max., 60 liters/hr
Thermization, pasteurization	APV Plate heat-exchanger-type paraflow Throughput max., 600 liters/hr for heating Jacketed vat, 500-liter capacity with stirrer and thermostatic control	Small-dimensioned plate heat exchanger with a corresponding lower throughput rate Jacketed vat, 50-liter capacity with stirrer and thermostatic control
Centrifugation for casein removal and final clarification	Alfa-Laval closed-bowl clarifier centrifuge, type K-2939 H Capacity of bowl, 20 liters Throughput max., 800 liters/hr	Westfalia closed-bowl centrifuge, type LG 205-8 Capacity of bowl, 0.3 liters Throughput max., 200 liters/hr
Ultrafiltration	DDS Module 35-18 Filtration surface, 18 m^2 Internal volume, 9 liters retentate Throughput, 170 liters permeate/hr Membrane type, GR81P	DDS Lab Unit 36–2.25 Filtration surface, 2.25 m^2 Internal volume, 1.13 liters retentate Throughput, 21 liters permeate/hr Membrane type, GR81P
Filtration for clarification and sterilization	Seitz filter holder, type A-207 with 9 20 × 20-cm plates	Seitz filter holder, type A-207 with 2 20 × 20-cm plates

TABLE 3. *(Continued)*

Procedure	Equipment used for 200–500 kg full cow's milk	Equipment proposed for 20–50 kg full human milk
	Filtration surface, 0.36 m²	Filtration surface, 0.08 m²
	Filtrox filter holder, type Econom with 7 40 × 40-cm plates	Millipore disk filter holder YY 30293 16 with MF-Filter HVLP
	Filtration surface, 1.12 m²	Filtration surface, 0.05 m²
	Millipore cartridge housing YY 14 131 00 with Millitube cartridge CEHA	
	Filtration surface, 0.12 m²	
Evaporation at low temperature	LUWA mechanically agitated thin film evaporator, type NL-150/1100/14	LUWA mechanically agitated thin-film evaporator, type L-82/500/14
	Heating surface, 0.5 m²	Heating surface, 0.125 m²
	Capacity, 50 kg water/hr	Capacity, 15 kg water/hr
Freeze-drying	Usifroid, model SM.I.R.	Usifroid, model SM.I.50.F.
	Ice capacity of condenser, 45 kg water	Ice capacity of condenser, 9 kg water

CONCLUSION

The procedures used in the isolation of a milk immunoglobulin concentrate from cow's milk could serve as a basis for the isolation of a protein isolate from human milk. Paradoxically, the introduction and realization of new procedures and isolation techniques are often linked to problems of "scaling up," but here we are faced with the necessity of "scaling down."

It is hoped that the procedures described in this chapter may assist in the work of supplementing pooled banked human milk with a standardized, immunologically active human milk protein isolate for the optimal nutrition of preterm and very-low-birth-weight infants.

REFERENCES

1. Chandra RK. Nutr Rev 1978;36:265–72.
2. Hambraeus L, Forsum E, Lönnerdal B. In: Food and immunology, Swedish Nutrition Foundation Symposium XIII. Stockholm: Almqvist and Wiksell International, 1977:116–24.
3. Mata L. Am J Clin Nutr 1978;31:2058–65.
4. Hibberd CM, Brooke OG, Carter ND, Haug M, Harzer G. Arch Dis Child 1982;57:658–62.
5. Rönnholm KAR, Sipilä I, Siimes MA. J Pediatr 1982;101:243–7.
6. Fomon SJ, Ziegler EE, Vasquez HD. Am J Dis Child 1977;131:463–7.
7. Raiha NCR. Pediatrics 1974;53:147–56.
8. Ziegler EE, Bigas RL, Fomon SJ. In: Suskind RM, ed. Textbook of pediatric nutrition. New York: Raven Press, 1981:29–39.
9. Lucas A, Gibbs JHA, Baum JD. Early Hum Dev 1978;2:351–61.
10. Lucas A, Lucas PJ, Chavin SI, Lyster RLJ, Baum JD. Early Hum Dev 1980;4:15–21.
11. Hilpert H, Gerber H, Amster H et al. In: Food and immunology, Swedish Nutrition Foundation Symposium XIII. Stockholm: Almqvist and Wiksell International, 1977;182–96.
12. Mietens C, Kleinhorst H, Hilpert H, Gerber H, Amster H, Pahud JJ. Eur J Pediatr 1979;132:239–52.

Human Milk Banking, edited by
A. F. Williams and J. D. Baum.
Nestlé Nutrition, Vevey/Raven Press,
New York © 1984.

Role of Nonantibody Proteins in Milk in the Protection of the Newborn

Bruno Reiter

National Institute for Research in Dairying, Shinfield, Reading RG2 9AT, England (retired) and Department of Pediatrics, University of Oxford, Oxford OX1 3PD, England

Since the turn of the century, the antibacterial activity of milk has attracted the attention of scientists in human and veterinary medicine. Medical workers were interested in the spread of milkborne diseases such as cholera, salmonellosis, and scarlet fever. Veterinarians researched the role of antibacterial factors in the defense of the bovine udder against bacterial infections (mastitis). Dairy scientists worried about the inhibition of lactic streptococci vital for the production of cheese.

Eventually, veterinarians discovered that ungulates are born without immunoglobulins in their blood and depend on the ingestion of colostrum and transmission of colostral antibodies through their permeable gut into the blood. An intestinal role for antibodies was proposed but could only be established after the discovery of secretory IgA. The attention of immunologists has been focused on the role of sIgA in defence against bacterial (and viral) intestinal infections in piglets, calves, and, more recently, human infants. This has resulted in the neglect of other host defense functions of human milk such as lysozyme, lactoferrin (transferrin), lactoperoxidase, etc. These factors can augment antibody action and afford protection in the absence or inefficiency of specific antibodies.

This chapter is concerned with the description, occurrence, and mode of action of these nonantibody factors *in vitro*. It also deals

29

with their *in vivo* activity insofar as the very limited range of animal experiments permit (for reviews, see 1–11).

LYSOZYME (N-ACETYLMURAMYLHYDROLASE, E.C. 3.2.1.17)

In 1922, Fleming (12) discovered the "extraordinary bacteriolytic phenomenon" of nasal mucus. He named the agent lysozyme. The wide distribution of lysozyme—in secretions such as milk, saliva, egg white, in tissue extracts (alveolar and intestinal), in "pus," and in blood—led him to believe that it constituted a primary method of destroying bacteria.

The concentration of lysozyme in human colostrum is relatively high (Fig. 1) (4); its concentration declines rapidly with the duration of lactation, but the increased intake of milk by the growing infant ensures an appreciable intake. However, relatively high levels are maintained through the first and possibly second year of lactation (13). In contrast, bovine milk contains little lysozyme (30 μg/100

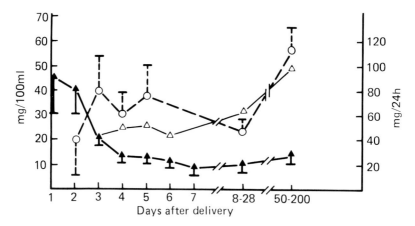

FIG. 1. Lysozyme in milk: concentration and daily intake. (▲) concentration (mg/100 ml) ± SEM; (○) intake (mg/24 hr) for group B subjects; (△) calculated intake (derived by multiplying milk volumes for group C by the mean concentration of lysozyme). Group B: milk samples provided daily and 24-hr test weighings at each sampling point. Group C: no analysis of milk samples, only 24-hr test-weighing data available. (From ref. 4.)

ml) (14). Unfortunately, we still lack sufficient *in vivo* evidence to substantiate that the relatively high concentration of lysozyme in human milk compared with bovine milk benefits the breast-fed infant.

Mode of Action and Antibacterial Spectrum

Lysozyme is a basic protein, stable at acid pH but unstable at alkaline pH. It hydrolyzes the β,1–4 linkage between N-acetylglucosamine in the peptidoglycan layer of the cell wall of gram-positive and the outer membrane of gram-negative organisms. The susceptibility of an organism to lysozyme depends on the accessibility of the substrate, peptidoglycan, and the origin of the enzyme. In gram-negative organisms, the susceptible substrate is masked by lipoproteins, hence the relative resistance to lysis unless the organisms are first exposed to the action of specific antibodies and complements or treated with agents such as chloroform or ethylenediamine-tetraacetic acid (15–17).

Human and bovine milk lysozymes (Tables 1, 2) have about three times the specific activity of egg albumen lysozyme as measured against the very susceptible assay organism *M. lysodeicticus*. The ease of purification of lysozyme from the enzyme-rich egg white and its commercial availability made this lysozyme regrettably the favorite tool for many investigations, notwithstanding the known differences between the lysozymes of different origins.

Biological Significance

Rosenthal and Lieberman (18) were the first to suggest in 1931 that lysozyme in human milk has a marked influence on the bacterial flora of the intestine in infants. They showed that the meconium contained no lysozyme; on the third day postpartum, the enzyme appears in the feces of breast-fed infants but not of artificially fed infants. The bacterial flora of the breast-fed infants was found to contain about equal numbers of gram-negative and gram-positive organisms. A suspension of such feces, incubated with complement-inactivated human milk for 24 hr at 37°C, contained few gram-

TABLE 1. *Sensitivity of different bacteria to human milk lysozyme[a]*

Organism	Rate of lysis (Δ% T/min)[b]
Streptococcus lactis	0.00
Staphylococcus aureus	0.05
Sarcine lutea	0.04
Streptococcus faecalis	0.04
Bacillus cereus	0.23
Escherichia coli	0.10
Serratia narcescens	0.00
Proteus vulgaris	0.00
Pseudomonas fluorescens	0.08
Pseudomonas aeruginosa	0.21
Micrococcus lysodeicticus	1.70

[a]Compiled from ref. 14.

[b]T is turbidity in phosphate buffer, pH 6.2, determined at 540 nm. For comparison, Δ% T/min for *M. lysodeicticus* by egg white lysozyme is 0.63.

TABLE 2. *Sensitivity of different bacteria to bovine milk lysozyme[a]*

Organism	Rate of lysis (Δ% T/min)[b]
Streptococcus lactis	0.2
Staphylococcus aureus	0.03
Sarcine lutea	0.08
Streptococcus faecalis	0.17
Bacillus cereus	0.10
Escherichia coli	0.12
Serratia marcescens	0.10
Proteus vulgaris	0.06
Pseudomonas fluorescens	0.08
Pseudomonas aeruginosa	0.30
Micrococcus lysodeicticus	1.82

[a]Compiled from ref. 14.

[b]T is turbidity in phosphate buffer, pH 6.2, determined at 540 nm.

negative organisms. When the feces were incubated with boiled human or raw cow's milk, they observed a relative increase in gram-negative organisms. The researchers attributed this effect of the human milk to its high lysozyme content and suggested that the enzyme may be an important factor in the welfare of infants. The main criticism of the inhibition experiments is that the antibacterial property of milk is now known to be multifactorial.

Recent work confirms the presence of lysozyme in the feces of breast-fed babies (19–21). The feces of infants with diarrhea contain more lysozyme than those of healthy infants. The increase of lysozyme in inflammatory intestinal mucosa parallels the immigration of neutrophilic leukocytes, monocytes, and macrophages, which release the enzyme into the intestinal fluid.

Besides the antibacterial properties of lysozymes, Jollès (22) proposed that lysozyme may have a function as an immunomodulator. Indeed, there exists some support for this hypothesis in the literature. Lodinová and Jouja (21) reported that a lysozyme-containing formula significantly increased the sIgA levels in the feces of full-term and preterm babies. The levels of IgM, IgG, and IgA in the serum were not increased. Because of the lack of humoral response, they suggested that the lysozyme activity on bacterial cell walls may stimulate a local immune response.

One may speculate further that the lysozyme content of milk promotes protection through its effect on human leukocytes. Human lysozyme at a concentration of 10 to 400 μg/ml significantly ($p < 0.001$) stimulates phagocytosis of yeast cells by leukocytes in the absence of any serum factors. Albumen lysozyme is without any effect. Lysozyme does not act on the yeast cells but on the leukocytes and cannot therefore be regarded as an opsonin (23).

LACTOFERRIN

The antibacterial activity of this iron-chelating protein was first reported in bronchial mucus and bovine milk (24–26). Lactoferrin has since been shown to be present in the milk of most mammals, albeit at different concentrations, and in the secretion of the nonlactating bovine mammary gland. The exception so far is rabbit's milk, which contains transferrin, the iron-binding protein in blood. Traces of transferrin are also found in most milks. Lactoferrin also occurs in other exocrine secretions such as saliva, tears, nasal, pancreatic, and intestinal secretions (27,28).

The concentration of lactoferrin (4) in colostrum (Fig. 2) is high, declining rapidly with postpartum age like lysozyme, but the total intake by the infant is considerable, remaining at around 1,000 μg/day for several weeks. Unlike lysozyme, lactoferrin has never been used as a supplement to formula feeds. However, a related protein, conalbumin, purified from egg white has recently been added with claims of a beneficial effect for infants with diarrhea.

Chemical Properties and Antibacterial Effect of Lactoferrin

Lactoferrin is a single-chain glycoprotein with a molecular weight of 70,000. It is strongly basic, binding two ferric ions and, syner-

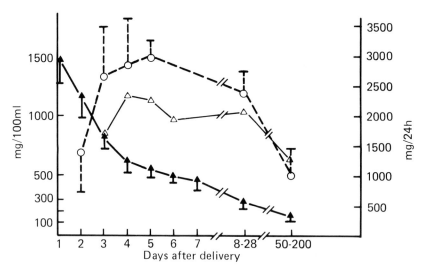

FIG. 2. Lactoferrin in milk: concentration and daily intake. (▲) concentration (mg/100 ml) ± SEM; (○) intake (mg/24 hr) for group B subjects; (△) calculated intake (derived by multiplying milk volumes for group C by the mean concentration of protein for each day). (From ref. 4.)

gistically, two bicarbonate ions; it holds iron at low pH (3.5–4), whereas transferrin loses its iron at low pH.

In the native state, lactoferrin is only partly saturated with iron (8–25%) and can therefore deprive bacteria of essential iron by its chelating power. It had been generally accepted (29–33) that only bacteria with a high iron requirement (e.g., coliforms) are inhibited, whereas organisms with very low iron requirements (e.g., lactic acid bacteria) (34) are not inhibited. Recent research has shown that a wide spectrum of bacterial species, both gram-positive and gram-negative bacteria, are not only inhibited but killed by apolactoferrin (devoid of iron), whereas the bacteriostatic activity of lactoferrin is only temporary and can be reversed by the addition of iron. The bactericidal activity of apolactoferrin is irreversible (35–38).

Although lactoferrin can withhold iron essential for the growth of organisms, the presence of citrate as in milk, 2 to 3 mM in human and 4 to 8 in mM in bovine milk, can make iron available for growth as an iron–citrate complex, which is taken up by bacteria. Bicarbonate, being essential for the chelating of iron by lactoferrin, can overcome this effect (39–42). Bacteria themselves also possess several means of iron chelation in an iron-poor medium or in the presence of lactoferrin: siderophores, siderochromes, secondary hydroxamic acids (e.g., ferrichromes, ferrioxamine B), and phenolic acids (e.g., enterocholin).

Bactericidal Effect of Apolactoferrin

Arnold and his collaborators (35–38) demonstrated in a series of papers that apolactoferrin (iron-free) in distilled water had a direct bactericidal effect on a wide range of microorganisms including gram-positive, gram-negative, aerobic, and anaerobic bacteria as well as yeast: *Streptococcus mutans, Streptococcus salivarius, Streptococcus pneumoniae, Escherichia coli* (nonenteropathogenic), *Vibrio cholerae, Pseudomonas aeruginosa, Candida albicans.* However, other morphologically and physiologically similar organisms are completely resistant: *Streptococcus pyogenes, Strep-*

tococcus lactis, Lactobacillus casei, Staphylococcus aureus, Staphylo-coccus epidermidis, Escherichia coli (0126,0111—enteropathogen-ic), Enterobacter cloacae, Salmonella newport, and Shigella sonnei.

The bactericidal effect, within 1 hr, cannot be reversed by iron or magnesium (known to stabilize the inner membrane) and is the result of a two-step process with a log phase of ~15 min. The apolactoferrin needs to remain in direct contact with the cell surface throughout. Viable organisms can be recovered after removal of the protein by washing within 50 min. Slime formation—S. mutans grown with sucrose—or capsule formation—S. pneumoniae pas-saged through an animal—reduces the bactericidal effect. The pro-cess is energy dependent: no killing occurs at 2°C, and organisms harvested in the early phase of stationary growth are markedly more resistant than organisms in the exponential phase. Detailed studies with S. mutans showed that glucose uptake and metabolism are inhibited, as is the incorporation of amino acids and purines.

So far there is no evidence that this bactericidal effect takes place in milk containing native lactoferrin; in vivo it may be of some relevance to the intracellular killing of leukocytes. The observed effect on the metabolism points to a damaging effect on the inner membrane remarkably similar to the effect of the lactoperoxidase system, which has been shown to damage the inner membrane. It is difficult to free all traces of lactoperoxidase from lactoferrin preparations (32). Also, since hemoproteins are known to have peroxidative activity, the bactericidal effect could be attributable either to this reaction or to contaminating lactoperoxidase.

Biological Significance

Human colostrum contains high concentrations of lactoferrin, up to 15 mg/ml; the concentration declines with postnatal age but less rapidly than those of sIgA, IgM, and IgG. However, with the increased intake of milk that occurs as the baby grows, the total intake of lactoferrin actually increases after birth and reaches a peak at about 5 days (4,13). This high intake suggests an important role for lactoferrin, but before we can ascribe a biological function, it has to be shown that lactoferrin escapes digestion and any detrimental effect of the low pH in the stomach. In general, human milk passes rapidly, "undigested," into the duodenum (43).

Samson et al. (44) submitted human colostrum to tryptic and peptic digestion *in vitro*: tryptic digestion failed to release the iron or abolish the bacteriostatic effect, but peptic digestion or keeping the colostrum at low pH abolished both properties. Indeed, keeping purified bovine lactoferrin at pH 5 or 3 leads to a loss of 25% or 90%, respectively, of its original iron-binding capacity, but this can be nearly restored by keeping the pH at 7.4 for 4 hr (32). These observations, plus the concentration of antitrypsin in milk, which remains relatively high up to 24 days post-partum (falling afterwards below the sensitivity of the assay used) (4), and rapid passage through the stomach indicate that lactoferrin may escape destruction at least in the early life of the newborn.

In Vivo Antibacterial Activity of Lactoferrin

The milk of guinea pigs is relatively rich in lactoferrin and transferrin (0.2–2 mg/ml of each). Bullen et al. (30) infected suckling guinea pigs orally with *E. coli* 0111 and killed some at daily intervals. The *E. coli* were colonizing both the small and large intestine, but gradually lactobacilli became the dominant flora within 3 to 5 days in the small intestine and within 3 days in the large intestine. In artificially fed piglets, the *E. coli* 0111 remained the dominant flora throughout, although lactobacilli began to establish themselves, particularly in the large intestine from 4 to 6 days. To prove that the iron-chelating proteins were responsible for the suppression of *E. coli*, a third group of suckling piglets were daily dosed orally with hematin; they were killed after 3 days only. Their intestines were predominantly colonized by *E. coli* 0111, although the large intestine already contained appreciable numbers of lactobacilli.

The suckled animals fed hematin showed an increase in *E. coli* of 4 log cycles in the small intestine and over 2 log cycles in the large intestine compared with the controls (suckled and no hematin)—obviously a striking difference. It is unfortunate that these piglets were killed after 3 days although all the other experiments lasted 6 days; even the artificially fed piglets began to be colonized by lactobacilli between 3 and 6 days (note that the lactobacilli appeared naturally).

The few *in vivo* experiments indicate that lactoferrin can contribute to the suppression of *E. coli* in the intestine. Large-scale experiments have so far been hindered because it proved impossible to develop a technological process to purify sufficient lactoferrin. Although bovine whey is in abundant supply, it contains only low concentrations of lactoferrin. An alternative source of an iron-chelating protein is egg white, which is rich in conalbumin; the antibacterial and iron-binding properties of conalbumins closely resemble those of lactoferrin (40,45,46).

At present, a number of clinical trials are being conducted with conalbumin. Infants with acute diarrhea have been fed formula and conalbumin, 600 to 1,200 mg/day. The therapeutic results appear to be promising (Table 3).

THE LACTOPEROXIDASE SYSTEM

The bactericidal property of milk was first recognized by Hesse in 1894 (48). Raw milk destroyed "cholerabacillus" within 12 hr at room temperature and within 6 to 8 hr at 37°C. Heating milk to 100°C destroyed this property. He suggested, therefore, that raw milk was not only unlikely to be a carrier for cholera bacilli but

TABLE 3. *Normalization of bowels of infants with acute enteritis (6 months to 1 year)[a]*

Treatment	3 days	3 to 6 days	6 to 9 days
Conalbumin (3.70 ± 0.36, n = 20)[b]	11 (55%)	7 (35%)	2 (10%)
No conalbumin (6.15 ± 0.41, n = 20)	1 (5%)	11 (55%)	8 (40%)

[a]U. Cornelli Ricordati (*personal communication*).
[b]$p < 0.01$ in favor of the group treated with conalbumin.

might be used as a prophylactic or therapeutic food. Hanssen (49) attributed the bactericidal power of milk against "bacillus typhosus and paratyphosus" to the peroxidative property of milk (measured by the color reaction with *para*-phenylendiamine in the presence of H_2O_2), which was destroyed by heating at 75°C for 15 min, as was the bactericidal activity. The bactericidal effect lasted only for 4 hr and varied according to season, with summer milk when the cows were on pasture being most effective. In retrospect, these observations describe unwittingly all three components of the lactoperoxidase (LP) system, consisting of lactoperoxidase, thiocyanate, and H_2O_2. Thiocyanate concentrations are high in the milk of cows on natural pasture (16), and freshly drawn milk probably contains some H_2O_2.

Eventually, lactoperoxidase was identified (50), the need for H_2O_2 established (51), and the third component identified as thiocyanate (52,53; for reviews see 5–7,9,11).

Distribution of the Components of the Lactoperoxidase System

Lactoperoxidase (LP, donor: H_2O_2 oxidoreductase, E.C. 1.11.1.7)

Lactoperoxidase is a trivial name derived from the source—milk—from which it had been first purified (54,55). It occurs not only in milk but also in saliva, tears, cervical mucus, and eosinophils. Their biochemical reactions—formation of complexes with H_2O_2 and oxidation of thiocyanate (SCN^-), bromide, and iodide—are identical. Lactoperoxidase consists of a single polypeptide chain with a molecular weight between 77,000 and 100,000; LPs derived from different organs in the same animal are immunologically identical.

Human milk has peroxidative bactericidal activity (11,56–58) (Fig. 3) largely derived from polymorphonuclear leukocytes (59). This enzyme is composed of two subunits, has a molecular weight between 118,000 and 144,000, and is not immunologically identical with LP; it also differs biochemically, because unlike LP it can also oxidize chloride. Although the peroxidative value of human milk is

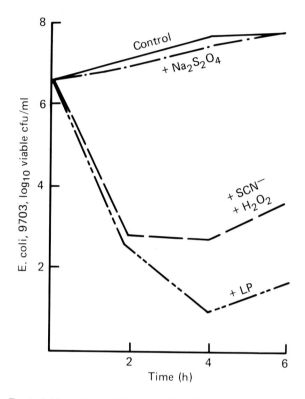

FIG. 3. Bactericidal effect of human milk (10 days after parturition) containing 20 mU ml⁻¹ LP. Control (—). Additions: SCN (0.225 nM) and H_2O_2 (0.222 mM) (- - -); as above plus 200 mU ml⁻¹ LP (- · · -); as above plus 1 mM $Na_2S_2O_4$ (- · · -). (From ref. 11.)

low, it must be remembered that the human infant is born with salivary LP that supplements the milk peroxidative activity.

An important characteristic of LP is its resistance to low pH and digestion. The peroxidative values of both bovine and human milk are preserved up to 2 hr in gastric juice from adults and infants with pyloric stenosis (56).

Thiocyanate

The thiocyanate anion (SCN⁻) (60–68) is highly permeable and thus ubiquitous in animal tissue and secretions. It is partly derived endogenously during the detoxification reaction between thiosulfate (metabolic produce of sulfur amino acids) and cyanide catalyzed by the liver and kidney enzyme rhodanase; principally, however, it is derived after ingestion of the anion, its esters, and other precursor compounds such as nitriles, isothiocyanates, and cyanide. Many plants are rich in glucosinolates (thioglycosides), which on hydrolysis by a thioglucosidase, myrosinase, yield SCN^- and/or isothiocyanate and nitriles. The *Cruciferae* are the most important source of thiocyanate for man and animals. Savoy kale contains from 85 to 500 ppm NaSCN, white cabbage about 32, cauliflower about 100, sauerkraut 33 to 200, and other vegetables from less than 1 up to 5 ppm. Some plants such as cassava, sweet potatoes, millet, sugar cane, bamboo, and lima beans are particularly rich in cyanogenic glucosides that, on hydrolysis, release considerable amounts of hydrogen cyanide, which is converted into thiocyanate. Tobacco smoke is also an indirect source of thiocyanate. The distribution of SCN^- in human plasma, saliva, gastric juice, urine, and milk is shown in Table 4. The anion occurs not only in biological secretions but also in synovial fluid, cerebrospinal fluid, and lymphocytes.

The concentration of SCN^- is influenced by the diet, at least in animals. The SCN^- content in bovine milk can be increased by feeding, for instance, kale (up to 13 ppm) or when the cows graze on natural pastures containing a varied flora (including clover, which contains cyanide). There are so far no data on whether the diet (or smoking) of the lactating mother influences the SCN^- content of her milk.

Hydrogen Peroxide

It is generally assumed that H_2O_2 is absent from milk. Theoretically, however, H_2O_2 can be generated by xanthine oxidase, sulfhydryl oxidase, or Cu^{2+} and ascorbic acid provided free O_2 is present.

Recently, we have shown (69) that milk leukocytes generate detectable amounts of H_2O_2 (nanomolar) in milk. Leukocytes phagocytize casein micelles (and fat globules) (70,71), a process that is known to produce an acceleration in metabolic activity generating

TABLE 4. *Concentration of thiocyanate (as ppm NaSCN) in human body fluids*[a,b]

Fluid	Nonsmoker	Smoker	Reference
Plasma	1.9 ± 0.74	6.7 ± 2.3	61
	(0.96–3.55)	(3.4–11.6)	
Saliva	37	155	62
Adults	73 ± 8	186 ± 32	65
	(19–60)	(58–270)	
Human infant	23 ± 15	—	56
Urine	16 ± 6	23 ± 11	
	(4–38)	(5–45)	
Gastric juice			
Fasting	73 ± 8		65
Stimulated	24 ± 3		
Milk	<6.5		56

[a]From B. Reiter, G. Mayntzan, and G. Härnulv (*unpublished*).
[b]Values are given as averages ± standard deviations (ranges in parentheses).

H_2O_2. Since milk contains both catalase and peroxidase, the H_2O_2 can only be detected after inactivation of the enzyme by sodium azide. *In vivo*, lactic acid bacteria are a source of H_2O_2. These organisms rapidly colonize the intestinal tract of newborns and are found to be H_2O_2 producing in the milk-fed calf (6,72). No data are so far available for the human newborn, but it can be expected that the same conditions prevail.

The Oxidation Products of Thiocyanate

Lactoperoxidase in the presence of H_2O_2 oxidizes SCN^- to a number of short-lived intermediate oxidation products with anti-bacterial activity (52,53). These are now recognized to be hypo-thiocyanite ($OSCN^-$), hypothiocyanous acid ($HOSCN^-$ at low pH), and higher oxyacids such as cyanosulfurous acid (H_2OSCN) and cyanosulfuric acid (H_3SCN); of these oxidation products, only $OSCN^-$ has been chemically synthesized. The end products of the oxidation are carbon dioxide, sulfate, and ammonia, all of which are inert, having no antibacterial effect (73). It has now been confirmed that the oxidation of SCN^- proceeds in stages of 1, 2, and 3 equivalents of H_2O_2, $OSCN^-$ being the first to appear (51,73–80). It has been suggested that $OSCN^-$ exerts the bacteriostatic activity and that the higher oxyacids are bactericidal for organisms such as *E. coli* (81) (Table 5). A recent detailed review of the interaction among LP, H_2O_2, and SCN^- has been published by Thomas (80).

The Mode of Action

Lactic acid bacteria that are catalase negative metabolize sufficient H_2O_2 under aerobic conditions to be inhibited in the presence of LP and SCN^- alone (52,53,73,75,83–85). Catalase-positive organisms such as coliforms, salmonellae, and shigellae, including multiple antibiotic-resistant strains, require an exogenous source of H_2O_2 (6,85–87) added as a chemical generated by an enzyme system such as glucose oxidase/glucose or in a mixed culture, where a surplus of H_2O_2 is produced metabolically. Although lactic acid bacteria (gram-positive) are only temporarily inhibited, gram-negative organisms are killed. Inhibition of streptococci affects growth, lactic acid production, and respiration; enzymes of the glycolytic pathway such as hexokinase are completely and glucose-6-phosphate dehydrogenase partly inactivated by the LP system. Some strains of the same species, however, can be completely resistant because they possess a "reversal factor" that reverses the inhibition of glycolysis (Fig. 4); this factor catalyzes the oxidation of $NADH_2$ in the

TABLE 5. *Oxidation of SCN⁻ by LP and H_2O_2[a]*

$H_2O_2 + SCN^-$	$\xrightarrow{\text{LP}}$	$OSCN^-$ [b] $+ H_2O$
$H_2O_2 + OSCN^-$	$\xrightarrow{\text{LP}}$	O_2SCN^- [c] $+ H_2O$
$H_2O_2 + O_2SCN^-$	$\xrightarrow{\text{LP}}$	O_3SCN^- [c] $+ H_2O$
End oxidation products: SO_4^{2-}, NH_4^+, CO_2		

[a]Compiled from refs. 60, 73, 75, 76, 81, 82.
[b]Bacteriostatic: $OSCN^- + R—SH \rightarrow R—S—SCN + OH^-$.
[c]Bactericidal.

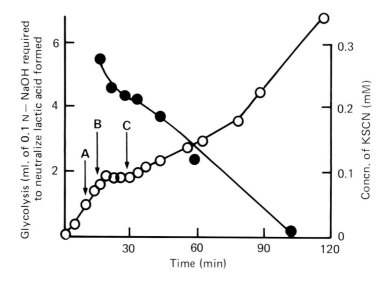

FIG. 4. Inhibition of the glycolysis of *Strep. cremoris* 972 by LP and KSCN and its reversal by an extract of *Strep. cremoris* 803. KSCN (5 μmoles) **(A)** and LP (70 units) **(B)** were added to a suspension of strain 972 in 0.1 M glucose, 10 mM potassium phosphate buffer, pH 6.8, and extract of strain 803 (1.0 ml) **(C)** was added later: (○) glycolysis; (●) concentration of residual KSCN corrected for volume changes. (From ref. 73.)

presence of an intermediate oxidation product of SCN⁻ [now assumed to be OSCN⁻ but then found to be mimicked by the chemically synthesized sulfurdicyanide S(CN)₂ (73)].

Both gram-positive and gram-negative organisms immediately leak potassium and amino acids, which indicates damage to the inner membrane. With gram-negative organisms such as coliforms or pseudomonads, this damage leads to death and eventually lysis (6,7,11). Why the leakage of gram-positive organisms does not lead to death is not clear. The lesser damage to the membrane indicated by lower leakage may be repairable; or the different composition and physical structure of the cell wall may act as a barrier (88). The damage to the inner membrane causes inhibition both of the uptake of nutrients such as glucose, amino acids, etc. and of the synthesis of protein, DNA, and RNA (1,84,89,90).

There are two aspects of the LP system that concern the attachment to brush borders and milk fat globules. It is generally agreed that certain potential pathogens attach themselves to the epithelial surface of the intestine. The intimate attachment favors proliferation of the organisms and reduces their removal within the lumen by peristalsis. Subsequently, enterotoxins are produced, which cause diarrhea. Specific sIgA prevents attachment and thus protects the infant.

When *E. coli* possesses K_{88} or K_{89} antigens, they attach to porcine or calf intestine, respectively, *in vivo*. Selwood et al. (91) developed an *in vitro* test whereby *E. coli* was found to attach specifically to the host brush border. When these organisms were treated with the LP system, they failed to attach to the brush border in the same number as untreated organisms. The LP system therefore had a similar effect to sIgA on attachment to the brush border (7,11). So far this phenomenon has not been confirmed *in vivo*.

Since fat globules are surrounded by a true cell membrane, we considered whether they have the same specific receptors as the brush border. Indeed, it was found that the enteropathogenic bovine strain of *E. coli* possessing K_{89} antigen only attached to bovine fat globule, and the porcine enteropathogenic strains possessing K_{88} antigen only to porcine fat globule. Human strains possessing either colonization factor CF1 or CF2 attached to human fat globule but also slightly to porcine fat. The bovine and porcine strains failed to attach to the same degree after treatment with the LP system. The human strains, however, remained unaffected (11). In this context, it is of interest that a high percentage of sIgA is attached to the fat globule membrane, incidentally proving that the level of sIgA in colostrum and milk may frequently have been underestimated (92). It remains to be seen whether the attachment of sIgA to fat globules has any significance for the protection of the newborn during the ingestion of the milk. Since it was suggested that the effect of the sIgA is to bind the organisms closer to the bacterial surface, it would therefore be interesting to test the LP system and sIgA for attachment.

Biological Significance of the LP System

According to the literature, human milk contains varying and small concentrations of peroxidase activity. If we accept that the peroxidative values represent cell-bound myeloperoxidase, we need to know whether the enzyme is released or not before and after ingestion. The contribution of the salivary LP during suckling appears to be important whatever the milk peroxidative values turn out to be. However, until we have more information available, we can only extrapolate from the results obtained with the calf. The advantages of using the calf as an experimental animal are that (a) it can be separated from the dam without ill effect; (b) as long as it is fed milk only, without any access to roughage, it remains a monogastric animal; (c) feeding host-specific milk avoids digestive and intestinal complications that arise by feeding, for instance, bovine milk to piglets or guinea pigs or infants; (d) it is relatively easy to cannulate the calf throughout the intestinal tract, and it grows slowly, thus allowing continuous experimentation.

We obtained some evidence that the LP system operates *in vivo* in the calf without an exogenous source of H_2O_2 (or SCN^-) (93–95) (Fig. 5). Calves were infected orally with *E. coli* as above and fed heated milk in which the LP had been inactivated (70°, 15 min). Nearly all the inoculum could be recovered from the abomasum when sampled at 30 min and 1 hr. Feeding raw milk reduced the number of *E. coli* by ~99%, indicating that the LP system was operating without the addition of an exogenous source of H_2O_2. The addition of a reducing agent restored the number of organisms to approximately the original inoculum. Complementing the raw milk with a source of H_2O_2, either glucose oxidase/glucose or magnesium peroxide, further reduced the number of *E. coli*; we assumed, therefore, that the calves were colonized by H_2O_2-producing organisms that activated the LP system. Indeed, it was found that >50% of the lactobacilli colonizing the intestinal tract produced H_2O_2.

Practical Application of the LP System

When calves are not reared on their dams but under prevailing commercial conditions, they are liable to scouring. Because of

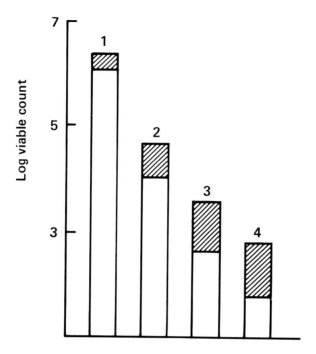

FIG. 5. Recovery of *E. coli* from abomasal fluid after feeding a cannulated calf with milk containing ~10^7 cfu/ml of *E. coli* *(1)* heated milk (no LP); *(2)* raw milk; *(3)* raw milk + GO/G; *(4)* raw milk + MgO₂; *(diagonal lines)* 30-min sample; *(open bars)* 1-hr sample. (From ref. 94.)

overcrowding and artificial feeding (powdered skim milk plus substitute fats), they are subject to bacterial (and viral) infections. We undertook large-scale trials involving some 300 animals to assess whether the LP system could ameliorate scouring caused by gram-negative potential pathogens and improve their performance measured according to their live weight gains. These trials lasted for 4 years (96).

In Sweden, calves were purchased from different farms 5 days after birth. It is known that the incidence of scouring is high under these circumstances. The calves were fed raw milk only and raw milk supplemented with glucose oxidase/glucose and SCN⁻ (at the time we had insufficient data about the likely concentration of SCN⁻ in the gastric juice). Although the days of scouring were only originally reduced from 3 days in the control animals to 2.3 days in the animals fed with the LP system, their live weight gain was 63% depressed during the first 3 weeks of the trial. In the following weeks, the difference in live weight gain diminished but was still 23% depressed over the whole 7 weeks of the experiment, after which the calves were weaned. In addition, the "LP calves" had a better appearance (sleek coat), were more lively, and consumed more solid supplement food.

The next three trials were performed at the National Institute for Research in Dairying; the calves were left for 2 days on the dam and then transferred to the calfhouse. Under these circumstances, the incidence of scouring was much less than in the purchased calves. The advantage of feeding the LP system was statistically significant for the first 5 weeks as measured by the live weight gain. Again, the number of days the animals scoured was reduced. The relationship between the percentage of animals scouring and the live weight gain is evident in Fig. 6. The more animals scoured, the higher the gains were to be expected by feeding the LP system.

The LP system has also been shown to be effective for the preservation of cooled and uncooled milk (94,97–99). Psycho-

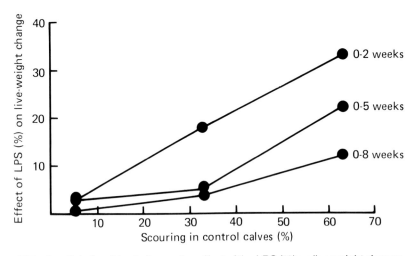

FIG. 6.   Relationships between the effect of the LPS (%) on live weight change and the level of scouring (%) in calves given whole milk only. (From ref. 96.)

trophic organisms multiplying at 4° to 10°, such as pseudomonads (gram negative), are inhibited for 3 days or more, thus preventing the spoilage of milk by their lipolytic and proteolytic activity. The shelf life of uncooled milk was increased by 6 to 12 hr in developing countries under ambient temperatures up to 37°C. Although the control milk (untreated) became quickly sour, the LP system suppressed the lactic acid formation sufficiently to preserve the milk (94).

CONCLUSIONS AND PROSPECTS

It is now generally accepted that colostrum and milk bridge the immunological gap in the newborn, thus protecting it against colonization of the intestinal tract by pathogens until the newborn builds up its own defense systems. The antibacterial activities of the nonantibody protective proteins and their mode of action have been well shown *in vitro*; there is, however, scanty documentation of their *in vivo* effects.

Since the milk of each species contains the nonantibody proteins in different concentrations and proportions, the effect of a single factor is difficult or impossible to determine when the newborn is allowed to suckle the dam. Ideally, we need to separate the newborn from the dam as early as possible, milk the dam, and, before feeding, treat the milk so that it contains only one protective protein or none for the control animals. This excludes the employment of conventional small laboratory animals: these are either too immature at birth, or it proves impossible to milk the dam. Alternatively, the newborn can be fed artificially with a formula feed supplemented with one of the protective proteins. Unfortunately, artificial feeding introduces another variant because the feeding of non-host-specific milk creates nutritional and digestive problems that can interfere with the interpretation of the experimental data.

The cannulated calf has proved to be well suited for the study of the lactoperoxidase system. However, a major difficulty in the use of calves or experimental animals is their high cost, elaborate housing, and attendance required. The miniature piglet may be better suited. The litters are large (average 6), and the piglets can be housed in cages and fed automatically. The milk could be obtained from conventional sows. Cannulation would be more difficult, but the large litter makes the piglets expendable.

The protective role of the LP system appears to be reasonably well established now in the calf, but its possible role in the human infant can only be surmised. Human milk does contain peroxidative activity, at least early in the lactation, but we need to know whether salivary LP supplements the lack of milk enzyme. Thiocyanate secretion occurs as early as the secretion of HCl, but how much do salivary LP and thiocyanate contribute to the gastric juice? The lactic acid bacteria colonizing mouth, esophagus, stomach, and upper duodenum generate H_2O_2. For this purpose, we need to obtain not only samples of saliva under different conditions but also intestinal samples.

Although the protective proteins may be of secondary importance for infants cared for under strict hygienic conditions, they may help to protect the low-birth-weight and premature baby. Research on the proteins may also lead to supplementation of baby feeds whenever breast feeding is not possible and help the development of a cheap antibacterial weaning feed. Such a feed would be helpful in developing countries, where intestinal infections are held down during breast feeding but can become endemic after weaning.

REFERENCES

1. Braun OH. Klin Paediatr 1976;188:297–310.
2. Goldman AS, Smith CW. J Paediatr 1973;83:1082–90.
3. Hanson LÅ, Winberg JW. Arch Dis Child 1972;47:845–8.
4. McClelland DBL, Grath J, Samson RR. Acta Paediatr Scand [Suppl] 1978;271:1–20.
5. Reiter B, Oram JD. Nature 1967;216:328–30.
6. Reiter B. In: Skinner FA, Hugo, WH, eds. Inhibition and inactivation of vegetative microbes. London: Academic Press, 1976:31–60.
7. Reiter B. Ann Rech Vet 1978;9:205–24.
8. Reiter B. J Dairy Res 1978;45:131–47.
9. Reiter B. In: Oxygen free radicals and tissue damage, Ciba Foundation Symposium No. 65 (new series). Amsterdam: Excerpta Medica, 1979:285–94.
10. Reiter B. In: Basselik-Chabielska L, ed. Resistance factors and genetic aspects of mastitis control. Jablonna, Poland: Ossolineum, 1980:351–391.

11. Reiter B. In: Lambert HP, Wood CBS, eds. Immunological aspects of infection in the fetus and newborn. London: Academic Press, 1981:155–95.
12. Fleming A. Proc R Soc (Lond) [Biol] 1922;93:306–17.
13. Goldman AS, Garza C, Nichols BL, Goldblum RM. J Pediatr 1982;100:563–7.
14. Vakil JR, Chandan RC, Parry RM, Shahani KM. J Dairy Sci 1969;52:1192–7.
15. Jollès P, Jollès J. Nature 1961;192:1187–8.
16. Osserman EF, Canfield RF, Beycho KS. Lysozyme. New York: Academic Press, 1974.
17. Witholt BW, van Heerikhuizen H, de Leij L. Biochim Biophys Acta 1976;443:534–44.
18. Rosenthal L, Lieberman H. J Infect Dis 1931;18:226–39.
19. Hanneberg B, Finne P. Acta Paediatr Scand 1974;63:588–94.
20. Isaacson P. Gut 1982;23:578–88.
21. Lodinová R, Jouja V. Acta Paediatr Scand 1977;66:709–12.
22. Jollès P. Biomedicine 1976;25:275–6.
23. Klockers M, Roberts P. Acta Haematol 1976;55:289–95.
24. Masson PL, Heremans JT, Prignot J, Wauters G. Thorax 1966;21:538–44.
25. Oram JD, Reiter B. Rep Natl Inst Res Dairy 1966:93.
26. Oram JD, Reiter B. Biochim Biophys Acta 1968;170:351–65.
27. Masson PL, Heremans JF, Schonne E. Clin Chim Acta 1966;14:735–9.
28. Masson PL. La Lactoferrine. Brussels: Arscia; Paris: Librarie Maloine, 1970.
29. Bullen JJ, Rogers HJ, Leigh L. Br Med J 1972;446:69–75.
30. Bullen JJ, Rogers HJ, Griffith E. Curr Top Microbiol Immunol 1978;80:1–36.
31. Fransson GB, Lonnerdal B. J Paediatr 1980;96:380–4.
32. Law BA, Reiter B. J Dairy Res 1977;44:595–7.
33. Weinberg ED. Microbiol Rev 1978;42:45–66.
34. Reiter B, Oram JD. J Dairy Res 1968;35:67–9.
35. Arnold RR, Cole MF, McGhee JR. Science 1977;197:263–5.
36. Arnold RR, Brewer M, Ganthier JJ. Infect Immun 1980;28:893–8.
37. Arnold RR, Russel JE, Champion WJ, Gauthier JJ. Infect Immun 1981;32:655–60.
38. Arnold RR, Russel JE, Champion WJ, Brewer M, Gauthier JJ. Infect Immun 1982;35:792–9.
39. Griffith E, Humphrey J. Infect Immun 1977;15:396–401.
40. Phelps CF, Antonini E. Biochem J 1975;147:385–91.
41. Reiter B, Brock JH, Steel ED. Immunology 1975;28:83–95.
42. Smith KL, Schanbacher FL. Am Vet Med Assoc 1977;170:1224–8.
43. Mason S. Arch Dis Child 1962;37:387–91.
44. Samson RR, Mirtle C, McClelland DBL. Acta Paediatr Scand 1980;59:517–23.
45. Antonini E, Orsi N, Valenti P. G Mal Infect Parasit 1977;2:481–9.
46. Schade AL. Biochem J 1963;338:140–4.

47. Valenti P, Destasio A, Seganti L, Mastromarino P, Sinibaldi L, Orsi N. J Clin Microbiol 1980;11:445–7.
48. Hesse W. Z Hyg Inpektr 1894;17:238–71.
49. Hanssen FS. Br J Exp Pathol 1924;5:271–80.
50. Wright RC, Tramer J. J Dairy Res 1957;24:174–83.
51. Jago GR, Morrison M. Proc Soc Exp Biol Med 1962;111:585–8.
52. Reiter B, Pickering A, Oram JD, Pope GS. J Gen Microbiol 1963;33:XII.
53. Reiter B, Pickering A, Oram JD. In: Molin N, ed. International Symposium, Food Microbiology 4th. Uppsala: Almqvist & Wicksell, 1964:297–305.
54. Morrison MH, Hamilton B, Stotz E. J Biol Chem 1957;228:767–76.
55. Morrison M, Allen PZ, Bright J, Jayosinghe W. Arch Biochem Biophys 1961;111:126–33.
56. Gothefors L, Marklund S. Infect Immun 1975;11:1201–15.
57. Spik G, Cheron A, Montreuil J, Dolby J. Immunology 1978;35:663–7.
58. Stephens S, Harkness RA, Cockle SM. Br J Exp Pathol 1979;60:252–8.
59. Moldoveano Z, Tenovuo J, Mestecky J, Pruitt KM. Biochim Biophys Acta 1982;718:103–8.
60. Aune TM, Thomas EL. Eur J Biochem 1977;80:209–14.
61. Ballantyne B. Clin Toxicol 1977;11:195–9.
62. Barylka-Pikielna N, Pangborn RM. Arch Environ Health 1968;17:739–43.
63. Moister FC, Freis ED. Am J Med Sci 1949;218:549–56.
64. Montgomery RD. Toxic constituents of plant food stuffs. In: Liener IE, ed. New York: Academic Press, 1969:143–57.
65. Ruddel WSJ, Blendis LM, Walters CL. Gut 1977;18:73–7.
66. Undritz E, Lang EM, van Oye E. Sang 1956;27:513–5.
67. Virtanen AI. Experientia 1961;17:1–11.
68. Wood JL. Chemistry and biochemistry of thiocyanic acids and its derivatives. In: Newman AA, ed. London: Academic Press, 1975:156–220.
69. Korhonen H. In: Bassalik-Chabielska L, ed. Resistance factors and genetic aspects of mastitis control. Warsaw: Ossolineum, 1981:421–40.
70. Russel MW, Reiter B. J Reticuloendothel Soc 1975;18:1–13.
71. Russel MW, Brooker BE, Reiter B. J Comp Pathol 1977;87:43–52.
72. Reiter B, Marshall VME, Philips SM. Res Vet Sci 1980;28:116–22.
73. Oram JD, Reiter B. Biochem J 1966;100:373–82, 382–8.
74. Adamson M, Pruitt KM. Biochim Biophys Acta 1981;658:238–47.
75. Hoogendoorn H, Piessens JP, Scholtes W, Stoddard LA. Caries Res 1977;11:77–84.
76. Pruitt KM, Tenovuo J. Biochim Biophys Acta 1982;704:204–14.
77. Pruitt KM, Tenovuo J, Andrews RV, McKane T. Biochemistry 1982;21:562–7.
78. Tenovuo J, Moldoveanu Z, Mestecky J, Pruitt KM, Rahemtulla BH. J Immunol 1982;128:726–31.
79. Thomas EL, Aune TM. Infect Immun 1978;20:456–63.
80. Thomas EL. In: Pruitt KM, Tenovua J, eds. The lactoperoxidase system: chemistry and biological significance. New York: Marcel Dekker (in press).
81. Björck L, Claesson O. J Dairy Sci 1980;63:919–22.
82. Hogg DM, Jago GR. Biochem J 1970;117:779–90 and 791–7.

83. Mickelson MN. J Gen Microbiol 1966;43:31–43.
84. Mickelson MN. J Bacteriol 1977;132:541–8.
85. Björck L, Rosén CG, Marshall VME, Reiter B. Appl Microbiol 1975;30:199–204.
86. Reiter B, Björck L, Marshall VME, Longman AG, Cousins CM. Ann Rep Natl Inst Res Dairying 1973/74:94.
87. Reiter B, Marshall VME, Björck L, Rosen C-G. Infect Immun 1976;13:800–7.
88. Marshall VME, Reiter B. J Gen Microbiol 1980;120:513–6.
89. Marshall VME, Reiter B. Proc Soc Gen Microbiol 1976;3:109.
90. Marshall VME. [Dissertation]. Reading: Reading University, 1978.
91. Sellwood R, Gibbons RA, Jones GW, Rutter JM. J Med Microbiol 1975;8:405–11.
92. Hill IR, Porter P. Immunology 1974;26:1239–50.
93. Reiter B, Hàrnulv BG. In: Proceedings T.D.F. Symposium. Kiel. Verlag Th. Mann, Gelsenkirchen-Buer 1981:50–3.
94. Reiter B, Hàrnulv BG. Dairy Ind Int 1982;(May):12–5.
95. Reiter B. In: Pruitt KM, Tenovua J, eds. The lactoperoxidase system: chemistry and biological significance. New York: Marcel Dekker (in press).
96. Reiter B, Fullford RJ, Marshall VME, Yarrow N, Ducker MJ, Knutsson M. Anim Prod 1981;32:297–306.
97. Björck L, Claesson O, Schulthess W. Milchwissenschaft 1979;34:726–9.
98. Harnùlv BG, Kandesamy C. Milchwissenschaft 1982;37:454–7.
99. Reiter B, Marshall VME. In: Russel AD, Fuller R, eds. Cold tolerant microbes in spoilage and environment. London: Academic Press, 1979:153–6.

Human Milk Banking, edited by
A. F. Williams and J. D. Baum.
Nestlé Nutrition, Vevey/Raven Press,
New York © 1984.

Preparation of Fat and Protein from Banked Human Milk: Its Use in Feeding Very-Low-Birth-Weight Infants

P. Hylmö, S. Polberger, I. Axelsson, I. Jakobsson, and N. Räihä

Nordreco AB, Bjuv, Sweden; and Department of Pediatrics, University of Lund, Malmö, Sweden

Current recommendations, both in Europe and the United States, emphasize breast feeding as the regimen of choice for the healthy term infant (1,2). However, there is still considerable debate in the pediatric literature about the nutritional adequacy of human milk for the preterm infant. Recent studies (3–5) have shown that moderately premature infants (31 to 36 weeks gestational age) attain intrauterine growth rates with adequate intakes of human milk, but the question of the nutritional requirements of the very-low-birth-weight infant still remains unanswered.

There is evidence that the requirements of the very small preterm infant for protein, energy, calcium, and sodium may be greater than can be provided by mature human milk alone. The recent findings that milk from mothers delivering preterm infants contains more protein, calories, and sodium than term milk also suggest this (6,7). However, in addition to being a source of nutrients, human milk also contains important nonnutritional components such as specific antiinfective factors, hormones, enzymes, and growth factors, which may be of great importance for the development of the very-low-birth-weight infant.

In order to initiate a controlled clinical study with the aim of defining the special nutritional requirements of the very-low-birth-

55

weight infant, we have designed a pilot plant to prepare fat and protein fractions from unpasteurized human donor milk. These fractions can be used for the enrichment of human milk. The overall aim of our studies is not simply to find an optimal nutritional supply for the very-low-birth-weight infant but also to supply the developing organism with the protective factors, growth modulators, enzymes, and hormones that are uniquely present in human breast milk. In this chapter, we describe the method used to prepare the cream and protein fractions and also present some preliminary analytical data on these milk fractions.

PILOT PLANT TECHNIQUE

Fat Separation

After gentle heating to ~50°C, the human milk was separated into skim milk and cream with an Alfa-Laval separator, LAPX 202. The separator was run at a speed of 7,000 rpm. The skim milk had a fat content of less than 0.5%, and the fat phase 50 to 60%. The cream was frozen in 5-g pellets and packed in vacuum.

Ultrafiltration

The equipment used was a DDS (Danish Sugar Industry) Lab module 20–072. The module has a filtration area of 0.72 m². The membrane used is of type GR 61 PP with a cut-off value of 20,000 (molecular weight).

The warm skim milk, 45 to 50°C, was immediately poured into a jacketed stainless steel tank. The tank was cooled by running cold tap water, 12°C, and within 10 min the milk reached room temperature, 15 to 20°C. In order to get sufficient permeate flow, the temperature was kept at 15 to 20°C. Lactose and water-soluble salts were separated from the milk by ultrafiltration. Small amounts of low-molecular-weight proteins were lost with the permeate.

Each cycle started with 15 liters of milk. About 12 to 13 liters of skim milk remained after fat separation. The ultrafiltration process was run for 6 to 8 hr in order to achieve the desired level of

demineralization and protein concentration. The permeate was replaced by cold tap water. A constant volume and viscosity of the
recirculating milk kept the permeate flow at a desirable high level.
Bacterial analysis of the final protein and fat preparations showed
acceptable quality.

Freeze-Drying

After ultrafiltration, the concentrate was freeze-dried. Freeze-
dried protein powder from 120 liters of human milk was mixed
thoroughly and packed into polyethylene-lined aluminum pouches
containing ~10 g each. A scheme for the technique used is shown
in Fig. 1.

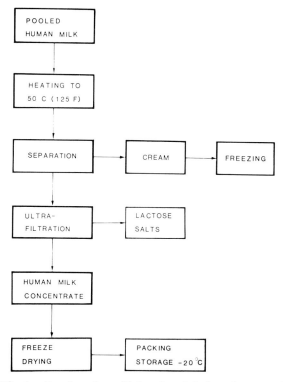

FIG. 1. Fractionation of fat and protein from human milk.

Preparation of Supplemented Human Milk

Supplemented milk is prepared for an infant freshly each day in a volume sufficient to last for 24 hr. The mother's own "raw" milk is preferentially used and is then complemented with banked milk to full volume. In general, the "mother's own" milk comprises ~30 to 50% of the total volume. When the mixture of "mother's own" and "pooled" milk is ready, it is supplemented with either protein powder or fat or both in amounts to make a total addition of 1 g protein and 1 g fat per 100 ml milk. This produces a final protein concentration of ~2 g/100 ml and a fat concentration of ~5.5 g/100 ml. The milk is then thoroughly mixed and divided into smaller plastic flasks, each containing the volume of milk needed for one feed. Samples for bacteriology and chemical analysis are taken from the supplemented milk. The criteria of acceptability are those currently employed by the milk bank.

PRELIMINARY ANALYSIS OF THE PROTEIN POWDER AND THE SUPPLEMENTED HUMAN MILK (HUMAN MILK FORMULA)

The crude protein powder contained 51% protein and 22.8% lactose (Table 1). When pooled human milk with a mean protein content of ~1 g/100 ml was supplemented with protein powder equivalent to 1 g of protein, there was a slight increase in the osmolality from 283 mOsm/kg to 290 mOsm/kg. Supplementation of the milk with fat produced no change in the osmolality (Table 2). There was no increase in sodium and potassium concentrations of the reconstituted human milk formula, but the calcium content rose by ~40% (Table 2) when protein was added.

In addition to the above assays, the milk protein powder was studied for the recovery of various whey proteins and enzyme proteins, which could theoretically be of advantage for the immature infant if administered in higher concentration than that present in pooled human milk.

Table 3 shows that the recovery in three separate production batches of α-lactalbumin, lactoferrin, lysozyme, and albumin varied

TABLE 1. *Protein and lactose in human milk protein powder*

Protein	51 g/100 g
Lactose	22.8 g/100 g

TABLE 2. *Osmolality and electrolytes in human milk preparations*

Preparation	Osmolality (mOsm/kg)	Na+ (mM)	K+ (mM)	Ca²⁺ (mM)
Human milk	283	7	16.4	7.7
Human milk + HM protein (1 g/dl)	290	8	16.5	10.9
Human milk + HM-fat (1 g/dl)	278	7	16.1	7.3

between 60 and 100%. Previous studies (8,9) have also shown a substantial recovery of lactoferrin and IgA in human milk protein preparations. The somewhat higher recovery in the present study was probably obtained because the protein powder was not pasteurized. Our human milk protein powder also contains activity of α_1-antitrypsin, amylase, and bile-salt-stimulated lipase (Table 3). Human milk bile-salt-stimulated lipase is readily inactivated when incubated at +50°C (10). In the present study, the low enzyme activity (15%) was apparently a result of the heating of the milk before the separation of the cream. In subsequent protein preparations, heating will be omitted in order to minimize the lipase inactivation. Almost 100% of the enzyme protein was, however, recovered in the human milk powder *(preliminary finding)*.

Clinical tolerance studies in very-low-birth-weight infants (<1,500 g body wt.) have shown that milk supplemented with 1 g of protein and/or 1 g of fat per 100 ml is well tolerated. Further controlled

TABLE 3. *Whey proteins and enzymes in human milk protein powder*

Component	Batch 1		Batch 2		Batch 3	
	Amount (mg/g)	Calculated recovery (%)[a]	Amount (mg/g)	Calculated recovery (%)	Amount (mg/g)	Calculated recovery (%)
α-Lactalbumin	100	80	—	—	90	94
Lactoferrin	60	60	100	100	12	70
Lysozyme	19	75	20	100		
Albumin	19	75	14	70		
sIgA	13.5	27	—	—		
α₁-Antitrypsin	0.34	28	0.34	28	0.7	87
Antichymotrypsin			0.0025	0.3	1.25	100
Amylase	160 (U/g)	100	180 (U/g)	100	270 (U/g)	100
Lipase	135[b]					

[a]Calculated recovery is expected recovery as related to fresh mature human milk.
[b]Expressed in micromoles of fatty acid released per gram per minute.

clinical studies are needed in order to evaluate the growth and metabolic effects of specially supplemented human milk in order to establish optimal feeding regimens for very-low-birth-weight infants. Such studies are currently in progress.

ACKNOWLEDGMENTS

These studies have been supported by funds from the Swedish Medical Research Council B82–19X-6259–01 and the Nestlé Nutrition Research Grant Programme. We would like to thank Dr. Lars Bläckberg, Umeå University, for the milk lipase assays.

REFERENCES

1. American Academy of Pediatrics, Committee on Nutrition. Pediatrics 1978;62:591–601.
2. ESPGAN Committee on Nutrition. Acta Paediatr Scand [Suppl] 1977;262:1–20.
3. Järvenpää AL, Räihä NCR, Rassin DK, Gaull GE. Acta Paediatr Scand 1983;72:239–43.
4. Järvenpää AL, Räihä NCR, Rassin DK, Gaull GE. Pediatrics 1983;71:171–8.
5. Rassin DK, Gaull GE, Järvenpää AL, Räihä NCR. Pediatrics 1983;71:179–86.
6. Atkinson SA, Bryan MH, Anderson GH. J Pediatr 1978;93:67–9.
7. Lemons JA, Moye L, Hall D, Simmons M. Pediatr Res 1982;16:113–7.
8. Lucas A, Lucas PJ, Chavin SI, Lyster RLJ, Baum JD. Early Hum Dev 1980;4(1):15–21.
9. Hagelberg S, Lindblad BS, Lundsjö A, et al. Acta Paediatr Scand 1982;71:597–601.
10. Hernell O. Eur J Clin Invest 1975;5:267–72.

Human Milk Banking, edited by
A. F. Williams and J. D. Baum.
Nestlé Nutrition, Vevey/Raven Press,
New York © 1984.

Growth Modulators in Human Milk: Implications for Milk Banking

Gerald E. Gaull, Charles E. Isaacs, Charles E. Wright, Leslie Krueger, and Harris H. Tallan

Department of Human Development and Nutrition, New York State Institute for Basic Research in Mental Retardation, Staten Island, New York 10314, U.S.A.

Milk is a complex fluid containing cells and membranes as well as a wide variety of soluble and insoluble components. Among the latter are the classical nutrients such as proteins and lipids (1). A puzzling aspect of the proteins is that the total protein content of human milk is the lowest among mammals. Indeed, it is not entirely clear how a normal breast-fed infant can grow so well on such small amounts of protein. On the other hand, there are a very large number of individual proteins in human milk as compared with the number of proteins found in a typical modern infant formula. A second major group of milk components consists of antiinfective or protective factors (2), the dominant one being sIgA. There is considerable evidence that these substances, protein in nature, are indeed protective against infection. Although most of the evidence has been obtained from studies *in vitro*, *in vivo* evidence in animal models (3) and prospective studies from developing countries give evidence of it also being true in man (4). A third group of constituents in human milk is beginning to be defined, i.e., growth modulators (Table 1). These are substances that can be shown to modify the growth and proliferation of cells. They include small molecules such as taurine (5), ethanolamine, and phosphoethanolamine (6) and small hormone-like proteins such as epidermal growth factor (EGF) (7) and nerve growth factor (NGF) (C. E. Wright and R.

TABLE 1. *Growth modulators in milk*

Nutrients
Amino acids (taurine)
Lipids (phosphoethanolamine, ethanolamine)
Minerals (Ca^{2+}, Cu^{2+}, Fe^{2+}, Se^{2+})
Vitamins (retinoids)
Hormones (insulin, thyroliberin, prolactin, endorphin)
Growth factors (epidermal growth factor, nerve growth factor)
Attachment factor (fibronectin)
Binding proteins (lactalbumin, transferrin, casein)
Polyamines (spermine, spermidine, putrescine)
Cells (B lymphocytes, T lymphocytes, macrophages, epithelial cells)
Others (interferon, drugs, environmental residues)

Rubenstein, *unpublished data*). Enzymes also may function in this capacity, although the evidence in this regard is unclear except for the lipases (8). Interferons have been identified in milk, which seem to be growth modulators as well as protective factors (9,10).

These constituents of milk are transferred from mother to off-spring during development, though the stage of development at which birth and nursing occur varies with the particular mammal. The purpose of this volume is to consider the role of human milk and formulas made from it in the feeding of the very-low-birth-weight infant, a relatively new biological entity whose viability is increasing along with advances in modern neonatology. This chapter is meant to draw attention to newly recognized growth modulators in human milk, which may interact with nutrients to "spare" them and, thereby, alter the baby's utilization and requirement for them. Any evaluation of milk banking and processing methods must take into consideration the possible effects of such procedures on these growth modulators.

GROWTH MODULATORS NEWLY RECOGNIZED IN HUMAN MILK

Assay of Growth Modulators by Cell Culture Systems

Cellular proliferation and differentiation constitute a complex process modulated by a finely balanced array of extracellular signals. Nutrients, hormones, and growth factors can initiate a myriad of biochemical reactions resulting in the growth and ultimate differentiation of cells. Cultured cells can grow in various media, which generally are supplemented with fetal bovine serum in order to maintain cell growth. Milk, however, also will promote the growth of cells. The growth of human fibroblasts on RPMI-1640 medium supplemented with 5% human milk is as good as that on medium supplemented with 5% fetal bovine serum. When the amount of human milk is increased, the growth of the fibroblasts is increased. When human milk is dialyzed to remove compounds with molecular weights $<10^4$, then the ability to support growth of fibroblasts is considerably reduced. These experiments show that, volume for volume, human milk supports dose-dependent growth of human cells as effectively as does the classical fetal bovine serum. Furthermore, a considerable amount of this growth effect is a function of molecules with molecular weights $<10^4$.

Taurine as a Growth Modulator in Human Milk

Taurine, 2-aminoethanesulfonic acid, is a small molecule of molecular weight 125. It may be a very "ancient" molecule, for it is among those substances synthesized under proposed primitive earth conditions (11). With regard to human milk, our interest in a possible role for taurine in infant nutrition began with the observation that preterm infants fed formulas had lower concentrations of taurine in their plasma and urine than similar infants nourished on human milk (12). This also has been shown to be true in the term infant (13). Taurine thus contrasts strikingly with most other amino acids, which usually have a higher concentration in the plasma of formula-fed infants. Some time ago, we established that taurine was the free amino acid present in highest concentration in human fetal brain during the second trimester (14), and we have since called attention to the potential role of taurine in development, as discussed in other reviews (15,16).

Recent experiments from our laboratory (17) have indicated that taurine has a proliferative effect on cultured human lymphoblastoid cells. This effect is maximal at 100 μM taurine in a chemically defined medium. At this concentration, the active transport system we have shown to be present in human lymphoblastoid cells (18) would be the major factor in taurine uptake, providing at least 90%, with diffusion accounting for <10%. It is of considerable interest that the concentration of taurine in the plasma of term infants is about 100 μM (13). Thus, uptake of taurine into cells and tissues, whatever its function, seems to depend in large part on the action of active transport systems similar to those found in human lymphoblastoid cells.

Although the growth effects of taurine in the cat (19) and in the monkey (20) are now well established, it has not been clear that growth effects are found in children. Indeed, in our recent studies of preterm infants (21), taurine seemed to have no effect on overall growth. However, there are now preliminary reports that severe and prolonged low plasma taurine concentrations in children with the blind-loop syndrome (22) or with prolonged total parenteral nutrition (23) can produce retinal damage similar to that seen in taurine-deficient cats. The retina, of course, is a tissue with a very rapid turnover of membranes, and there is increasing evidence that taurine is involved in the stabilization of certain cellular membranes (24).

In summary, taurine acts in the manner of a growth factor, as do its structural analogs ethanolamine and phosphoethanolamine (6). It may be a primitive growth factor. From the point of view of feeding the very-low-birth-weight infant, the point to be made is that presently available synthetic formulas contain very little taurine, but it is present in considerable concentrations in human milk (25). Fortunately, there are no problems with solubility or stability.

Protein Growth Modulators in Milk

The list of potential milk-associated growth modulators is large, but the list of confirmed modulators found in milk is small (Table 1), and their physiological functions in the neonate are not well defined.

Recent evidence has demonstrated that human milk contains several proteins that promote growth of cultured cells; the major protein resembles epidermal growth factor (EGF) (26,27). In addition, using cell culture and immunological assays, we have recently demonstrated that human milk contains nerve growth factor (NGF) (C. E. Wright and R. Rubenstein, *unpublished data*). In man, both EGF and NGF have not been characterized precisely, but both have been well characterized in the mouse (26,28). Both have been detected in nanogram per milliliter concentrations in murine milk. Murine EGF and NGF are present in high concentrations in the submaxillary gland and saliva of adult male mice; EGF is the most potent stimulator of epidermal and epithelial tissue growth and differentiation, whereas NGF is essential for the survival and development of sympathetic and some sensory neurons. Salivary EGF and NGF are passed into the gastrointestinal tract. Although EGF is present in gastric secretion in a biologically active form, it is not known whether this is also true of NGF. The presence of these growth factors in the saliva of adult mice, their complete absence from the salivary glands and saliva of suckling mice, and their presence in milk suggest that milk may be providing substantial amounts of these growth factors essential for specialized growth and maturation of various target tissues in the suckling neonate. Thus, it is possible that milk in the neonate is substituting for the salivary source of these components found in the adult.

The mere presence of both factors in the milk does not define their physiological function in the neonate. One can only speculate on possible roles. For example, EGF could function in the maturation of the epithelium of the immature gastrointestinal tract or could support the rapid growth and differentiation of epithelial cells in other tissues, especially the liver. Since EGF inhibits the release of gastric acid, it might also regulate pH in the stomach of the neonate (26). After birth, NGF may be involved in the arborization of sympathetic neurons in the gut or in the maturation of sensory neurons. Until these possible functions are elucidated, it would be prudent to assume these proteins to be active and to try to preserve them during milk banking procedures.

OTHER MODULATORS NEWLY RECOGNIZED IN HUMAN MILK

Enzymes in Human Milk

There are at least 60 to 70 enzymes in human milk, some of which are control-point enzymes for major metabolic pathways, e.g., glucose-6-phosphate dehydrogenase. Little is known, however, about their *in vivo* function. At least one human milk enzyme, bile-salt-stimulated lipase, has been shown to be active in the intestine and to play a physiological role in the digestion of milk triacylglycerols (29,30). It is unlikely, considering the strict control of secretory processes (31), that most enzymes occur in milk simply because of "spillage" from the blood or acinar cells.

Sulfhydryl oxidases (SOX) are a class of enzymes originally found in bovine milk (32) that catalyze the net synthesis of disulfide bonds using low-molecular-weight thiols or proteins as substrates *in vitro*. The *in vivo* substrates of sulfhydryl oxidases found in mammalian secretions and tissues have not been established. We have performed experiments to determine whether or not SOX and other human milk enzymes have characteristics similar to those of other milk proteins, e.g., sIgA and lactoferrin, which have been shown to be active in the gastrointestinal tract.

Sulfhydryl oxidase is present in the milk of all species that have been studied (human, bovine, rat, rabbit, rhesus monkey, and macaque). Human milk SOX is very stable in an acid environment: no activity is lost at pH 4.0; 75 to 80% of the activity remains at pH 3.0; and >50% remains at pH 2.5. Human milk SOX is not inactivated at pH 11. Human milk SOX is also resistant to gut proteases. After exposure to 4,000 units of pepsin for 90 min *in vitro*, human milk SOX retains 40 to 45% of activity. Sulfhydryl oxidase is also relatively resistant to trypsin and to chymotrypsin but not to the combination. Since human milk SOX has a pH optimum between 7.0 and 7.5, it apparently could function in the small intestine after passage through the stomach. The human milk γ-glutamyltranspeptidase (GGT) is also acid stable, and >70% of its activity remains after 1 hr at pH 4.0.

Pasteurization (62°C for 30 min) inactivates only 25% of bovine milk SOX activity, but human milk SOX is completely inactivated. However, 65% of activity remains after treatment at 60°C for 10 min. Relative heat stability is also characteristic of other milk proteins that have been shown to function in the gastrointestinal tract, e.g., sIgA and lactoferrin. We have shown that SOX, GGT, lactate dehydrogenase, and alkaline phosphatase from rat milk are stable in the stomach of suckling 7- to 9-day rats. Measurements of the contents of the proximal small intestine indicate that active SOX and GGT pass from the stomach to the intestine (33).

Milk enzymes may function in the milk itself, in the gastrointestinal tract (e.g., altering the mucin diffusion barrier), in the intestinal tissue, or may be absorbed by the proximal small intestine and transported to other target tissues. In a mouse plasmacytoma, SOX is known to be involved in the assembly of IgM. Thus, as with growth modulators it may be prudent to attempt to retain the activity of these enzymes under milk-banking and processing conditions.

Interferons in Human Milk

Interferons are a family of glycoproteins consisting of approximately 20 members (34). They have been shown to mediate a number of biological states, including host defense, growth, and immunocompetence. Human infants are known to be deficient in the mitogen-induced immune (Class II) interferon (35). It is of interest, therefore, that interferons are found in milk and milk cells (36,37). In light of their known antiviral and antiproliferative activities, it is possible that they may have an effect on the health and well-being of infants. The potential *in vivo* effect of maternal interferons has been assessed by us in a cell culture model. A proliferating human lymphoblastoid line dependent on the addition of 2% pooled human milk has been established. When interferon is added to this culture system, the interferon is biologically as active or more active than with control cells grown in serum. These preliminary results indicate that interferon added to human milk remains active in the initiation of the antiviral and growth modulatory states and suggests that endogenous interferons are similarly active.

CONCLUSIONS

The functions for these milk-associated growth modulators are potentially of considerable importance to the neonate. Two-dimensional gel examination of human milk proteins suggests that we have recognized the activity of only a few growth modulators. Until their roles *in vivo* are defined or can be dismissed as inconsequential, care should be taken to preserve them in human milk-banking procedures.

ACKNOWLEDGMENTS

Studies from the authors' laboratories were supported by the New York State Office of Mental Retardation and Developmental Disabilities and, in part, by NIH, NCI grant 1PO CA 29545.

REFERENCES

1. Gaull GE, Jensen RG, Rassin DK, Malloy MH. In: Milunsky A, Friedman EA, Gluck L, eds. Advances in perinatal medicine, vol 2. New York: Plenum Press, 1982:47–120.
2. Kraehenbuhl JP, Bron C, Sordat B. Curr Top Pathol 1979;66:105–57.
3. Schafer TW, Lieberman M, Cohen M, Came PE. Science 1972;172:1326–7.
4. Narayanan I, Prakash K, Baba S, Verma RK, Gujurol VY. Lancet 1980;2:561–3.
5. Gaull GE, Wright CE, Tallan HH. In: Iwata H, Kuriyama K, Huxtable R, eds. Proceedings, international symposium on sulfur amino acids. New York: Alan R. Liss, Inc., 1983;257–303.
6. Murakami H, Masui H, Sato GH, Sueoka N, Chow TP, Kano-Sueoka T. Proc Natl Acad Sci USA 1982;79:1158–62.
7. Carpenter G. Science 1980;210:198–9.
8. Shahani KM, Kwan AS, Friend BA. Am J Clin Nutr 1980;33:1861–8.
9. Bocci V. Biol Rev 1981;56:48–85.
10. Borden EC, Ball LA. Prog Hematol 1981;12:299–339.
11. Choughuley ASU, Lemmon RM. Nature 1966;210:628.
12. Gaull GE, Rassin DK, Räihä NCR, Heinonen K. J Pediatr 1977;90:348–55.
13. Järvenpää A-L, Rassin DK, Räihä NCR, Gaull GE. Pediatrics 1982;70:221–30.
14. Sturman JA, Gaull GE. J Neurochem 1975;25:831–5.
15. Gaull GE, Rassin DK. In: Meisami E, Brazier MAB, eds. Neural growth and differentiation. New York: Raven Press, 1979;461–77.
16. Sturman JA, Rassin DK, Gaull GE. Life Sci 1977;21:1–22.

17. Wright CE, Schweitzer LB, Gillam BM, Tallan HH, Gaull GE. J Pediatr Gast Nutr (in press).
18. Tallan HH, Jacobson E, Wright CE, Schneidman K, Gaull GE. Life Sci 1983;1853–1860.
19. Hayes KC, Carey RE, Schmidt SY. Science 1975;188:949–51.
20. Hayes KC, Stephan ZF, Sturman JA. J Nutr 1980;110:2058–64.
21. Järvenpää A-L, Räihä NCR, Rassin DK, Gaull GE. Pediatrics 1982;70:214–20.
22. Sheikh K. Gastroenterology 1981;80:1363.
23. Geggol HS, Ament ME, Heckenlively JR, Kopple JD. Clin Res 1982;30:486A.
24. Gaull GE, Sturman JA, Wen GY, Wisniewski HM. In: Hoffman JF, Giebisch GH, Solis L, eds. Membranes in growth and development. New York: Alan R. Liss, 1982:349–55.
25. Rassin DK, Sturman JA, Gaull GE. Early Hum Dev 1978;2:1–13.
26. Carpenter G, Cohen S. Annu Rev Biochem 1979;48:193–216.
27. Klagsbrun M. Proc Natl Acad Sci USA 1979;75:5057–61.
28. Greene LA, Shooter EM. Annu Rev Neurosci 1980;3:353–402.
29. Hernell O, Olivecrona T. Biochim Biophys Acta 1974;369:234–44.
30. Jensen BG, Clark RM, deJong FA, Hamosh M, Liao TH, Mehta NR. J Pediatr Gast Nutr 1982;1:243–55.
31. Mellman I. Nature 1982;299:301–2.
32. Janolino VG, Swaisgood HE. J Biol Chem, 1975;250:2532–8.
33. Isaacs CE, Pascal T, Wright CE, Gaull GE. Pediatr Res 1984;18:532–535.
34. Lengyel P. Annu Rev Biochem 1982;51:251–82.
35. Bryson YJ, Winter HS, Gard SE, Fischer TJ, Stiehm ER. Cell Immunol 1980;55:181–200.
36. Keller MA, Kidd RM, Bryson YJ, Turner JL, Carter J. Infect Immun 1981;32:632–6.
37. Lawton JWM, Shortridge KF, Wong RLC, Ng MH. Arch Dis Child 1979;54:127–30.

Human Milk Banking, edited by
A. F. Williams and J. D. Baum.
Nestlé Nutrition, Vevey/Raven Press,
New York © 1984.

Cloning Proteins from Human and Guinea Pig Milk

Roger K. Craig, Len Hall, Michael S. Davies,
and Peter N. Campbell

*Courtauld Institute of Biochemistry, The Middlesex Hospital Medical School,
London W1P 7PN England*

Although the main theme of this volume includes the composition of human milk and the specific requirements for different components of milk for infant nutrition, our interest in milk proteins has been generated for rather different reasons. For a number of years we have been interested in the many complex intracellular mechanisms involved in the expression of structural genes in higher organisms. The lactating mammary gland provides an attractive system for a variety of reasons.

Early studies based on antibody precipitation procedures using antibodies raised against mainly rat, rabbit, or mouse milk proteins demonstrated that milk protein gene expression was modulated by an intricate combination of steroid and peptide hormones (1), although the precise intracellular mechanism of action of these hormones remained to be established. With the development of techniques for the rapid isolation of eucaryote mRNA and the identification of mRNA species by cell-free protein synthesis, interest in the intracellular mechanisms involved in the synthesis of mammalian proteins increased. Invariably, studies were based on those systems in which a few well-defined proteins were produced in response to specific hormonal stimuli. Consequently, as the milk proteins fall into this category, the manner in which they are synthesized and secreted by the cells of the mammary gland has important implications for biology far beyond their basic relevance to lactation.

We are using the lactating guinea pig mammary gland as an animal model system with which to study gene structure, transcriptional and posttranscriptional mechanisms (2–5), and processes within the secretory pathway required for the sequestration and post-translational modification of proteins destined for secretion (6–9). Our interest in human milk protein gene expression stems from observations that suggested, on the basis of immunoassay procedures, that milk proteins, in particular α-lactalbumin, might prove a useful marker for the diagnosis of hormone-responsive human breast cancer (10–13), though the application of highly sensitive molecular techniques has since proven these hopes to be unfounded (14).

In general terms, the major milk proteins may be loosely classified into those that are acid precipitable, the caseins, and those that remain acid soluble, the whey proteins. Guinea pig milk contains three major casein components (A, B, and C) of estimated MW 28,000, 25,000 and 20,500 as determined by SDS–polyacrylamide gel electrophoresis (15). In common with all other caseins examined (16), guinea pig caseins are phosphoproteins and contain typically high concentrations of glutamic acid and proline but no cysteine. Human milk contains two caseins, the major component, MW 25,000, and a minor component, the k-casein. Both human and guinea pig milk contain a single predominant whey protein, α-lactalbumin. Human and guinea pig α-lactalbumins, MW 14,500, have been purified, and their primary amino acid sequences determined (17,18). Interest in α-lactalbumin has been considerable because of its role in the synthesis of lactose (19,20) and because of the suggestion that the structurally related but functionally distinct proteins α-lactalbumin and lysozyme have arisen from a common ancestral gene (21).

The prerequisite for any studies on the structure of milk protein genes, the intracellular mechanisms involved in mRNA biosynthesis, protein synthesis, or to a lesser extent secretion of the synthesized protein requires that an intact mRNA preparation be isolated from fresh or frozen mammary tissue and that the resulting mRNA population be shown to contain milk protein mRNA species. We have isolated total poly(A)-containing RNA from essentially normal human lactating mammary tissue (2 g retention cyst) obtained from a nursing mother 15 days post-partum (13). Addition of this to a wheat germ cell-free system in the presence of ^{35}S-methionine resulted in the net incorporation of ^{35}S-methionine into proteins over the endogenous background. Analysis of the *in vitro* synthesized ^{35}S-labeled protein products using SDS–polyacrylamide gel electrophoresis and visualization of the synthesized products by fluorography revealed the presence of three prominent bands of estimated molecular weights 26,500, 23,000, and 16,500 (Fig. 1). However, none of these products coelectrophoresed with the authentic human milk proteins (casein 25,000; lactalbumin 14,500), a situation similar to the mRNA-directed synthesis of guinea pig milk proteins in the wheat germ cell-free protein-synthesizing system. Product analysis using a mixture of antibodies raised against highly purified preparations of the major human casein component and of human α-lactalbumin resulted in the preferential precipitation of all three bands, whereas treatment with antisera raised against α-lactalbumin alone resulted in the precipitation of the lowest molecular weight component only.

These results are consistent with the synthesis in the wheat germ cell-free system of a precursor form of α-lactalbumin (pre-α-lactalbumin) and probably two precursor forms of human casein. We have purified and raised antisera against the high-molecular-weight casein, although it is known that this cross reacts immunologically

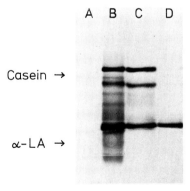

A B C D

Casein →

α-LA →

FIG. 1. Polyacrylamide gel electrophoresis of human milk proteins synthesized *in vitro* in a wheat germ system: *(A)* no added mRA; *(B)* total protein synthesized; *(C)* proteins synthesized and reacting to antibody to total milk proteins; *(D)* as in *C* but antibody specific to human α-lactalbumin; *(Arrows)* positions of authentic mature proteins isolated from human milk.

with the k-casein component (11). Thus, it seems reasonable to conclude that both bands represent human caseins and that the higher-molecular-weight predominant protein probably represents a precursor to the major human casein, whereas the minor lower-molecular-weight protein probably represents the equivalent precursor to the k-casein.

The anomalous electrophoretic mobility of the primary translation products of human and guinea pig milk proteins reflects the absence in cell-free systems of intracellular membrane-associated processing and posttranslational modification mechanisms, integral components of the secretory pathway (22). Thus, milk proteins in common with most proteins destined to be secreted are synthesized *in vitro* with nascent NH_2-terminal "signal" peptide extensions (23) (see also Fig. 4). *In vivo*, the interaction of the signal peptide (in combination with other protein factor; 24,25) with the endoplasmic reticulum results ultimately in the segregation of the secretory protein within the lumen of the endoplasmic reticulum, the first step of the secretory process, and also the removal of the signal peptide. Gel analysis of the casein primary translation products is further complicated by the absence of phosphorylation *in vitro* (26), since the enzyme responsible is an integral membrane protein associated with the Golgi apparatus of the mammary gland and so absent from the cell-free system (8).

Isolation and characterization of total poly(A)-containing RNA encoding milk proteins provided the basis of subsequent experimentation involving recombinant DNA technology designed to determine the nucleotide sequence of mRNA species encoding the individual milk proteins and, ultimately, the means to identify and characterize the genomic DNA sequence encoding the individual milk protein genes and flanking regulatory sequences. The techniques and strategies used for cloning mRNA populations have been reviewed at length (27,28). Briefly, a double-strand cDNA population representative of the total poly(A)-containing RNA isolated from lactating guinea pig or human mammary tissue was inserted into the plasmid pAT153 using A:T homopolymer tailing as outlined in Fig. 2 (see refs. 29,30 for a detailed description). The resulting

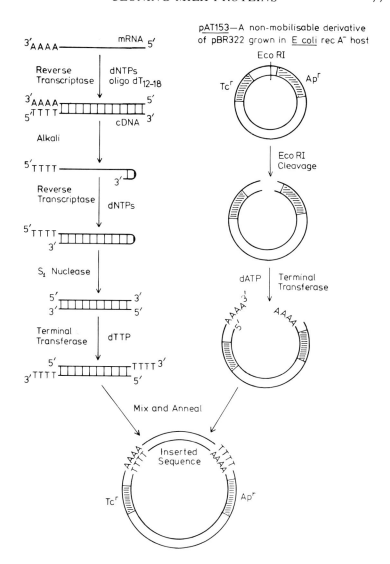

FIG. 2. Construction of recombinant DNA molecules containing milk protein mRNA sequences.

library of bacterial colonies was then screened in a preliminary manner by *in situ* hybridization using the appropriate ^{32}P-labeled lactating mammary gland mRNA as the hybridization probe as a means to select colonies containing recombinant plasmids representative of the most abundant (milk protein) mRNA sequences. Selected colonies were grown in bulk, the plasmid DNA isolated, and the cloned cDNA sequence within each plasmid identified by positive hybridization translation (hybridization of individual mRNA to immobilized recombinant plasmid DNA and subsequent identification of the selected mRNA by cell-free translation). For example, four recombinant plasmids isolated from a lactating guinea pig mammary gland cDNA library, pgp N-33, pgp K-27, pgp O-22, and pgp K-9, could be shown to hybridize mRNA encoding precasein A, B, and C and pre-α-lactalbumin, respectively (Fig. 3).

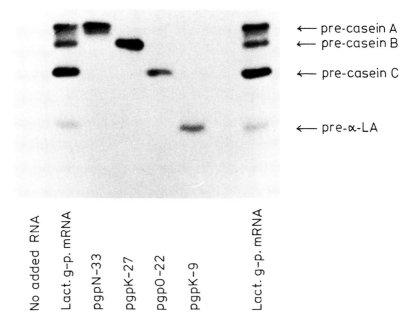

FIG. 3. Identification of recombinant plasmids containing guinea pig milk protein cDNA sequences by positive hybridization–translation.

Ultimate proof that the selected plasmids contain the desired cDNA sequence requires DNA sequence analysis and then selection of the appropriate reading frame by alignment of amino acid sequences deduced from the genetic code with known amino acid sequences. Using the DNA-sequencing procedure of Maxam and Gilbert (31), we have determined the nucleotide sequence of the human and guinea pig α-lactalbumin mRNA species by sequencing the cloned cDNA (32).

This has proved revealing in several senses (see Fig. 4). Comparison of the deduced amino acid sequences with the published sequences of human (18) and guinea pig (17) α-lactalbumins isolated from milk confirms that both are synthesized as precursor proteins with characteristic NH$_2$-terminal extensions as previously indicated by cell-free protein synthesis (see Figs. 1 and 3). The signal sequences in common with those of other known secretory proteins are rich in nonpolar hydrophobic amino acids (33) required for interaction of the nascent polypeptide with protein factors prior to interaction with the endoplasmic reticulum (24,25).

Examination of the nucleotide-deduced amino acid sequence of the 123 residues comprising the mature human and guinea pig α-lactalbumins (as found in milk) confirms the reported protein sequencing data (17,18) except for discrepancies between glutamic acid and glutamine or aspartic acid and asparagine residues. Although the human nucleotide sequence has a termination codon (TGA) at the expected position immediately after residue 123, the guinea pig sequence derived from the recombinant plasmid pgpK-9 does not. Instead, there is a CGA codon (Arg) at this position, the first termination signal being 37 codons downstream, suggesting a 36-amino-acid extension after the expected carboxyl-terminal glutamine residue. Analysis of five other plasmids containing guinea pig α-lactalbumin cDNA sequences derived from the same cDNA library and four other plasmids containing human α-lactalbumin sequences all revealed a termination codon (TGA) in the expected position immediately following residue 123. Interestingly, it has recently been reported that rat α-lactalbumin has a 17-residue carboxyl-terminal extension as revealed by cDNA sequence analysis

Human   5'
Guinea-Pig 5' GGTAAACTAGGGTAGCATAGGGAAGAGGGGTTCTGGGTGTATGGAAGAGCACGGGCATTTCAGGTTCACAGCAGCAGCCAAA

```
                                          700 .
Human       ATG AGG TTC TTT GTC CCT
Guinea-Pig  ATG ATG TCC TTT TTC CCT
            Met Arg Phe Phe Val Pro
                Met Ser       Phe
            -19 -18 -17 -16 -15 -14
```

```
                                                        600.
Human       CTG TTC CTG GTG GGC ATC CTG TTC CCT GCC CTG AAG CAA TTC ACA AAA AAA TGT GAG CTG TCC CAG CTG CTC AAA GAC ATA GAT GGT TAT
Guinea-Pig  CTG TTG CTG GTG GGC ATC CTT CCT GCC CTG GTG CAG CAA CTT ACC AAA     TGT GGG TCT GAG CTG CTG AAC TTG AAG GAC GAC GCC GGC TAC
                Leu                                 Val Gln           His Glu                           Asn         Ala
            Leu Phe Leu Val Gly Ile Leu Phe Pro Ala Ile Leu Ala Lys Gln Phe Thr Lys Cys Glu Leu Ser Gln Leu Leu Lys Asp Ile Asp Gly Tyr
            -13 -12 -11 -10 -9  -8  -7  -6  -5  -4  -3  -2  -1   1   2   3   4   5   6   7   8   9  10  11  12  13  14  15  16  17  18
```

```
            .                           500 .                               .             .   .
Human       GGA GGC ATC GCT TTG CCT GAA ATG TTT CAC ACC AGT GGT TAT GAC ACA CAA GCC ATA GTT GAA AAC AAT GAA AGC ACG AAA GAA
Guinea-Pig  CGA GAC ATC ACT TTG CCT GAA TGG CTC ATA TTT CAT ATC AGT GGT TAT GAC ACA ACA GCC ATA GTG AAA AAT AGT GAC CAC AAA GAG
            Arg Asp         Thr         Trp Leu     Ile Ile                     (Asp Gln)              Ser Asp His
            Gly Gly Ile Ala Leu Pro Glu Leu Cys Ile Thr Met Phe His Thr Ser Gly Tyr Asp Thr Gln Ala Ile Val Glu Asn Asn Glu Ser His Lys Glu
            19  20  21  22  23  24  25  26  27  28  29  30  31  32  33  34  35  36  37  38  39  40  41  42  43  44  45  46  47  48  49
```

```
            .   .                   .   .   :   :           .   :   :   :                           .                       .
Human       TAT GGA CTC TTC CAG ATC CTC AAT AAG CTT TGG TGC AAG AGC AGC CAG GTC CCT CAG TCA AGG AAC ATC TGT GAC ATC TCC TGT GAC AAG TTC
Guinea-Pig  TAC GGA CTT TTC CAG ATA CTT AAT GAT AAA GAT TGC TGT GAC AGC AGC GTC ACG CAA GTT ACT TCA AGG AAC ATT AAC TGT GAC ATT TCC GAC AAG CTC
                                        Asn Asp Asp     Asp Phe     Thr Thr Val                         (Asn)                   Glu              Leu
            Tyr Gly Leu Phe Gln Ile Leu Asn Lys Leu Trp Cys Lys Ser Ser Gln Val Pro Gln Ser Arg Asn Ile Cys Asp Ile Ser Cys Asp Lys Phe
            50  51  52  53  54  55  56  57  58  59  60  61  62  63  64  65  66  67  68  69  70  71  72  73  74  75  76  77  78  79  80
```

```
 400
CTG GAT GAT GAC ATT ACT GAT GAC ATA ATG TGT GCC AAG AAG ATC CTG GAT ATT AAA GGA ATT GAC TAC TGG TTG GCC CAT AAA GCC CTC TGC
CTG GAT GAT GAC CTT ACT GAT GAC ATA ATG TGT GTC AAG AAG ATC CTG GAT ATC AAA GGA ATT GAC TAC TGG TTG GCC CAC AAA CCA CTG TGC
   (Asn)   (Asn)       (Asn Asn)                                                 (Asn)
Leu Asp Asp Asp Ile Thr Asp Asp Ile Met Cys Ala Lys Lys Ile Leu Asp Ile Lys Gly Ile Asp Tyr Trp Leu Ala His Lys Ala Leu Cys
                Leu                         Val                                                                 Pro
81  82  83  84  85  86  87  88  89  90  91  92  93  94  95  96  97  98  99  100 101 102 103 104 105 106 107 108 109 110 111
   (Asn)   (Asn)       (Asn Asn)                                                 (Asn)

                    300
ACT GAG AAG CTG GAA CAG TGG CTT TGT GAG AAG TTG TGA GTG TCT GCT GTC CTT GGC ACC CCT GCC CAC TCC ACA CTC CTG GAA TAC CTC TTC
TCT GAC AAG CTG GAG CAG TGG TAC TGC GAG GCA CAG CGA GCA CCT GAT GTA TCT GCC AAT CCT GCT CTT CCC ATA CAC CCA GAA CCC CTC TTC

Thr Glu Lys Leu Glu Gln Trp Leu Cys Glu Lys Leu Stop
Ser Asp                     Tyr         Ala Gln Arg Ala Pro Asp Val Ser Ala Asn Pro Ala Leu Pro Ile His Pro Glu Pro Leu Phe
112 113 114 115 116 117 118 119 120 121 122 123 +1                          +10

                            200
CCT AAT GCC ACC TCA GTT TGT TTC TTT CTG TT CCC CCA AAG CTT ATC TGT CTC TGA GCCTTGGGCCCTGTAGTGACATCACCGAATTCTTGAAGACTATTTTCC
CCT CAT GCT ACC CCA GTT TAC CTT TTT CTG — CCC CTG AAT ATG ATT TGT CTC TGA GCCTTGGATCCTGTAGTGACACTGTTTGGCTCTTGAGGACTGTTGTCT

Pro His Ala Thr Pro Val Tyr Leu Phe Leu    Pro Leu Asn Met Ile Cys Leu Stop
+20                                        +30             +36

             100
AGGGATGCCTGAGTGGTGCACTGAGCTCTAGACCCTTACTCAGTGCCTTCGATGGCACTTTCACTACAGCA-CAGATTTCACCTCTGTCTTGAATAAAGGTCCCACTTTGAAGTC poly(A)
AAGGATGCATGACTGGTGCACTGGACATTAGAC——ACTCAGTGCCCTTGA————ACTACACCAACAAATCCCACTTCTGTCCTGAATAAAGGCCCTGATTTGG  poly(A)
```

FIG. 4. Nucleotide sequence of mRNA species encoding guinea pig and human α-lactalbumin.

(34), although in this instance all 14 α-lactalbumin clones examined were identical. The biological significance of a proline-rich hydrophobic extension has yet to be established. It is possible that α-lactalbumin has an additional intracellular role, presumably related to glycosylation events, in which the hydrophobic carboxyl-terminal extension is required to anchor the functional part of the protein to a membrane component within the secretory pathway. The existence of such a sequence would imply either multiple α-lactalbumin genes or alternative RNA splicing patterns (35).

Comparison of the nucleotide sequence within the coding region of the human and guinea pig α-lactalbumin mRNA demonstrates a high degree of homology, which extends to the coding region of chick lysozyme mRNA, observations that support the initial hypothesis based on amino acid sequence alone that lysozymes and α-lactalbumins evolved from a common ancestral gene (32). The construction and sequencing of cloned α-lactalbumin and lysozyme cDNA from other species will extend these studies and enable predictions to be made as to the time scale involved in evolutionary terms at which the divergence of α-lactalbumin and lysozyme genes occurred as a result of gene duplication.

In conclusion, the advent of recombinant DNA technology has provided the ability to investigate the structure and expression of mammalian genes and will ultimately provide insight into their regulation by hormonal stimuli. Moreover, via the construction of mutant genes coupled to recombinant constructions capable of expressing the encoded protein, it will provide a means of examining the relationship between protein structure and function. The technology will also permit the characterization of minor components of milk present in insufficient amounts to be examined by classical protein sequence analysis.

ACKNOWLEDGMENTS

We are grateful to Mr. M. R. Edbrooke and Mr. D. Parker for valuable technical assistance, and we acknowledge the financial support of the Cancer Research Campaign, the Medical Research Council, and the Wellcome Trust.

REFERENCES

1. Craig RK, Campbell PN. In: Larson BL, ed. Lactation: a comprehensive treatise vol IV. New York: Academic Press, 1978:387–404.
2. Bathurst IC, Craig RK, Campbell PN. Biochem J 1979;181:501–4.
3. Bathurst IC, Craig RK, Herries DG, Campbell PN. Eur J Biochem 1980;109:183–91.
4. Craig RK, Bathurst IC, Herries DG. Nature 1980;288:618–9.
5. Burditt LJ, Parker D, Craig RK, Getova T, Campbell PN. Biochem J 1981;194:999–1006.
6. Craig RK, Brown PA, Harrison OS, McIlreavy D, Campbell PN. Biochem J 1976;160:57–74.
7. Craig RK, Boulton AP, Harrison OS, Parker D, Campbell PN. Biochem J 1979;181:737–56.
8. Pascall JC, Boulton AP, Craig RK. Eur J Biochem 1981;119:91–9.
9. Pascall JC, Boulton AP, Parker D, Hall L, Craig RK. Biochem J 1981;196:567–74.
10. Woods KL, Cove DH, Howell A. Lancet 1977;2:14–6.
11. Laurence DJR. Invest Cell Pathol 1978;1:5–22.
12. Kleinberg DL, Todd J. Cancer Res 1978;38:4318–22.
13. Hall L, Craig RK, Campbell PN. Nature 1979;277:54–6.
14. Hall L, Craig RK, Davies MS, Ralphs DNL, Campbell PN. Nature 1981;290:602–4.
15. Craig RK, McIlreavy D, Hall RL. Biochem J 1978;173:633–41.
16. Jenness R. In: Larson BL, Smith VR, eds. Lactation: a comprehensive treatise, vol III. New York: Academic Press, 1974:3–107.
17. Brew K. Eur J Biochem 1972;27:341–53.
18. Findlay JBC, Brew K. Eur J Biochem 1972;27:65–86.
19. Brodbeck V, Ebner KE. J Biol Chem 1966;241:762–4.
20. Brew K, Vanaman TC, Hill RL. Proc Natl Acad Sci USA 1968;59:491–7.
21. Brew K, Vanaman TC, Hill RL. J Biol Chem 1967;242:3747–9.
22. Palade G. Science 1975;189:347–58.
23. Blobel G, Dobberstein B. J Cell Biol 1975;67:835–51.
24. Walter P, Blobel G. J Cell Biol 1981;91:557–61.
25. Meyer DI, Krause E, Dobberstein B. Nature 1982;297:647–50.
26. Mercier JC, Gaye P. Ann NY Acad Sci 1980;343:232–51.
27. Williams JG. In: Williamson R, ed. Genetic engineering, vol 1. London: Academic Press, 1981:1–59.
28. Craig RK, Hall L. In: Williamson R, ed. Genetic engineering, vol 4. London: Academic Press 1983;58–125.
29. Craig RK, Hall L, Parker D, Campbell PN. Biochem J 1981;194:989–98.
30. Hall L, Davies MS, Craig RK. Nucleic Acids Res 1981;9:65–84.
31. Maxam AM, Gilbert W. Methods Enzymol 1980;65:499–560.
32. Hall L, Craig RK, Edbrooke MR, Campbell PN. Nucleic Acids Res 1982;10:3503–15.

33. Steiner DF, Quinn PS, Chan SJ, Marsh J, Tayer HS. Ann NY Acad Sci 1980;343:1–16.
34. Dandekar AM, Qasba PK. Proc Natl Acad Sci USA 1981;78:4853–7.
35. Amara SG, Jonas V, Rosenfeld MG, Ong ES, Evans RM. Nature 1982;298:240–4.

Human Milk Banking, edited by
A. F. Williams and J. D. Baum.
Nestlé Nutrition, Vevey/Raven Press,
New York © 1984.

Studies on Nonimmunoglobulin Inhibitory Activity in Human Milk Against *E. coli* Heat-Labile Enterotoxin, Rotavirus, and Respiratory Syncytial Virus

*Anne-Brit Kolstø Otnæss, *Astrid Lægreid,
†Ivar Ørstavik, and *Karin Trollerud

Vaccine Department, National Institute of Public Health; and †Microbiological Laboratory, Ullevål Hospital, Oslo, Norway

It is well known that human milk will protect infants against various gastrointestinal infections (1,2). Colostrum and milk contain several components that are thought to contribute to this protective function (3,4). The single most important component is probably secretory IgA. The secretory IgA antibodies of the milk, which are considered not to be absorbed into the infant's circulation, have specificities against common enteric pathogens and are thought to play a local protective role in the infant's intestine. Although the relative importance of nonimmunoglobulin antiinfectious components of the milk is not known, these components are likely to be of greatest importance when the specific antibody to the infectious agent is at low concentration in the milk.

In our studies we have focused on the nonspecific inhibitory activity of human milk against *E. coli* heat-labile enterotoxin (LT) and rotavirus, which are two agents known to cause serious diarrhea in infants. We have also studied respiratory syncytial virus (RSV), since this agent is known to cause serious illness in the lower respiratory tract, and breast feeding has been reported to have a protective effect against it (5).

MATERIALS AND METHODS

Human milk was collected from healthy women from 3 days to 8 months post-partum. The milk was centrifuged (20,000 × g for 2 hr), and the milk fat and skimmed milk were analyzed separately. The milk cells at the bottom of the centrifuge tubes were discarded. The skimmed milk was fractionated by ammonium sulfate precipitation and column chromatography as described previously (6). The milk fat was extracted by chloroform and methanol and submitted to solvent partition (7) as described (8), followed by gel filtration in organic solvent (8,9).

The enterotoxin inhibitory activity was measured as the inhibition of toxin binding in the enzyme-linked immunosorbent assay (ELISA) (6,10). Since cholera toxin and *E. coli* heat-labile enterotoxin (LT) are very similar, and antiserum raised against one toxin will neutralize the other toxin, we used anticholera toxin in the ELISA. Briefly, microtiter plates were coated with anticholera toxin or with the ganglioside G_{M1} (11), and aliquots of LT preincubated with milk fractions or with buffer were added to the plate. In the next step, anticholera toxin produced in rabbits was added, followed by antirabbit immunoglobulin produced in swine and coupled to alkaline phosphatase. Inhibitory activity in the milk fractions caused a reduced color development of the substrate *para*-nitrophenylphosphate, and the yellow color was read in an eight-channel photometer. Alternatively, the inhibitory activity of the milk fractions was measured *in vivo* in rabbit intestinal loops (12) using several dilutions of cholera toxin (13).

The rotavirus inhibitory activity was measured as specific antibodies with immunofluorescence (IFA) or ELISA as described (10,14) and by virus neutralization test as described by Thouless et al. (15) with slight modifications (14).

Virus-specific IgA and neutralizing activity in the milk fractions against RSV were measured by indirect immunofluorescence and by virus neutralization, respectively (A. Lægreid et al., *unpublished data*). The inhibitory effect was measured by adding dilutions of milk fractions and virus to monolayers of LLC MK2 cells and incubating for 1 hr, and, after removal of the nonadhered virus, the cells were incubated overnight. The cells were fixed in methanol, and the monolayer stained for RSV by an indirect immunofluorescence test.

RESULTS AND DISCUSSION

Enterotoxin Inhibitory Activity

When measured by ELISA, all milk samples so far investigated (>100) inhibited the *E. coli* LT, but there was a considerable variation in inhibitory activity from one sample to another. In colostrum samples, 70 to 100% of the toxin was inhibited, whereas the values for late milk were somewhat lower (40–100%). Inhibitory activity was found in both skimmed milk and milk fat (Table 1). The inhibitory activity in skimmed milk had an apparent molecular weight greater than 400,000 (6), and the fact that it could be extracted from purified fractions of the skimmed milk by chloroform and methanol indicated that it was of lipid nature (10). The inhibitory activity was isolated from the milk fat by chloroform and methanol extraction; the ganglioside fraction of the milk fat inhibited the fluid accumulation in *in vivo* experiments with enterotoxin in rabbit intestinal loops (8,13). Further purification of the milk

TABLE 1. *Inhibition of* E. coli *LT by milk and milk fractions*

	Percent inhibition of LT measured by ELISA			
	Human milk	Cow's milk	Nestlé formula milk	Collett formula milk
Uncentrifuged milk	100	90	80	70
Skimmed milk	80	60	60	40
Milk fat[a] (0.1 g milk fat/ml)	90	80	80	60

[a]The milk fat was extracted with chloroform and methanol and partitioned for the isolation of gangliosides. After evaporation to dryness, the samples were dissolved in a volume corresponding to 0.1 g milk fat/ml.

ganglioside indicated that the toxin inhibitory activity had a structure very similar to the ganglioside G_{M1} (8); G_{M1} is known to be the receptor structure for cholera toxin and *E. coli* LT on the cell surface (21), and it thus appears that the toxin inhibitory activity of the milk may be similar to the toxin receptor. Milk ganglioside is likely to be in the fat fraction as well as in the skimmed milk, where it is probably associated with the milk fat globule membranes with an apparent molecular weight >400,000. It remains to be seen whether the inhibitory activity described by Holmgren and coworkers (17) is part of the inhibitory structure we have described.

Enterotoxin inhibitory activity was measured in cow's milk and milk formulas by ELISA. Inhibitory activity was present, although reduced when compared to human milk (Table 1). This difference is more pronounced in the case of colostrum. The cow's milk and the milk formulas were centrifuged, and the fat fractionated. Toxin inhibitory activity was observed in the ganglioside fractions, although the activity appeared lower in one of the milk formulas (Table 1). The exact nature of the ganglioside inhibitory activity in human and cow's milk and in milk formula is currently being studied.

Rotavirus Inhibitory Activity

Human milk contains both specific antibodies to rotavirus and an inhibitor of nonimmunoglobulin nature (14,15). When samples of colostrum from Ethiopian and Norwegian women were compared, similar amounts of both the specific antibodies and the nonspecific inhibitory activity were observed (10) (Table 2) in spite

TABLE 2. *Effect of milk on rotavirus*

Milk	n	Specific IgA		Rotavirus neutralization
		IFA	ELISA	
Ethiopian	14	1.3 (0–4)	34 (<8–128)	18.8 (<5–≥40)
Norwegian	11	1.5 (0–4)	28 (<8–128)	18.6 (<5–≥40)

of the fact that Ethiopian women may be more exposed to rotavirus infections as a result of their living conditions. Totterdell et al. (18) concluded that factors other than rotavirus antibodies are probably of importance in preventing infection. The nonimmunoglobulin inhibitor of rotavirus was trypsin sensitive with an apparent molecular weight <50,000 (10). The extracted milk fat did not inhibit rotavirus; this activity is, therefore, different from the lipid antiviral activity described by Welsh et al. (19).

Respiratory Syncytial Virus Inhibitory Activity

Virus-specific IgA was present in very few samples and at very low titers. Only mature milk samples were analyzed (1–8 months post-partum). Neutralizing activity was detected in a higher number of samples. After fractionation of the skimmed milk by ammonium sulfate treatment, virus-neutralizing activity was present in both the IgA-enriched and the IgA-poor milk fractions (Table 3). The IgA-poor fractions were further submitted to column chromatography, and the apparent molecular weight of the inhibitor was found to be >150,000. When the active fractions were pooled and passed through an anti-IgA affinity column, virus inhibitory activity was retained, indicating that the inhibitory activity was nonimmunoglobulin in nature. These RSV-neutralizing fractions did not neutralize rotavirus. In preliminary experiments, no RSV inhibitory activity was detected in cow's milk or milk formulas. The inhibitory factor will be further purified and characterized, and its activity measured against other respiratory viruses.

Our results are in agreement with those of Toms et al. (20), who reported that RSV-neutralizing activity persisted longer through lactation and at a higher titer than RSV-specific IgA. Transplacentally acquired IgG gives no or at best very poor protection at mucosal surfaces. Although the RSV-specific IgA titer is low in mature milk, it is often high in colostrum, and the bronchomammary axis may be of great importance in the immune response to RSV (16).

TABLE 3. *RSV-specific IgA and RSV inhibition of human milk fractions after ammonium sulfate treatment*

Sample No.	IgA-poor milk fraction			IgA-enriched milk fraction		
	sIgA (g/liter)	RSV-specific IgA titer	RSV neutralization titer	sIgA (g/liter)	RSV-specific sIgA titer	RSV neutralization titer
1	0.07	<2	<5	7.2	2	20
2	0.9	<2	<5	5.0	<2	5
3	0.01	<2	<5	5.0	<2	<2
4	1.0	<2	20	2.5	<2	20
5	0.1	<2	20	3.6	<2	20
6	0.6	<2	20	7.3	<2	20
7	0.1	<2	5	0.9	<2	5
8	0.07	<2	20	1.2	<2	20
9	0.3	<2	<5	1.5	<2	<2
10	3.5	<2	10	9.7	<2	5
11	1.0	2–4	>5	6.4	4	5
12	<0.01	<2	<5	2.4	<2	80
13	0.08	<2	<5	4.0	<2	5
14	1.3	<2	40	19.2	2	40
15	0.3	2–4	5	3.6	32	80
16	0.08	<2	<5	8.0	<2	20
17	0.01	<2	<5	1.4	<2	<5

CONCLUSIONS

Human milk contains inhibitory activity of nonimmunoglobulin nature against *E. coli* heat-labile enterotoxin and cholera toxin, and it may contain nonimmunoglobulin inhibitory activity against rotavirus and respiratory syncytial virus. The enterotoxin nonimmunoglobulin inhibitory activity is similar to G_{M1}, which is the receptor for the toxin, whereas milk lipid fractions show no neutralizing activity against the virus. The rotavirus-neutralizing factor is trypsin sensitive with an apparent molecular weight $<50,000$. The respiratory syncytial virus-neutralizing factors have an apparent molecular weight $<150,000$. The enterotoxin inhibitory activity was also detected in cow's milk and milk formula but was less than that observed in human milk.

Although the relative importance of these inhibitory components in human milk is not yet understood, their role should be considered in the feeding of infants.

ACKNOWLEDGMENTS

This work was supported by the Norwegian Research Council for Science and Humanities, by the Diarrhoeal Diseases Control Programme of the World Health Organization, and by the Norwegian Association Against Asthma and Allergies.

REFERENCES

1. Gerrard JW. Pediatrics 1974;54:757–64.
2. Larsen SA, Homer DR. J Pediatr 1978;92:417–8.
3. Goldman AS, Smith CW. J Pediatr 1973;82:1082–92.
4. McClelland DBL, McGrath JJ, Samson RR. Acta Pediatr Scand [Suppl] 1978;271:1–20.
5. Pullan CR, Toms GL, Martin AJ, Gardner PS, Webb JKG, Appleton DR. Br Med J 1980;281:1034–6.
6. Otnæss A-B, Halvorsen S. Acta Pathol Microbiol Scand [C] 1980;88:247–53.
7. Svennerholm L, Fredman L. Biochim Biophys Acta 1980;617:97–107.
8. Kolstø Otnæss A-B, Lægreid A, Ertresvåg K. Infect Immun 1983;40:563–569.
9. Siakotos AD, Rouser G. J Amer Oil Chem Soc 1965;42:913–9.
10. Otnæss A-B, Ørstavik I. Infect Immun 1981;33:459–66.

11. Svennerholm A-M, Holmgren J. Curr Microbiol 1978;1:19–23.
12. Svennerholm A-M. Int Arch Allergy Appl Immun 1975;49:434–52.
13. Otnæss A-B, Svennerholm A-M. Infect Immun 1982;35:738–40.
14. Otnæss A-B, Ørstavik I. Acta Pathol Microbiol Scand 1980;88:15–21.
15. Thouless ME, Bryden AS, Flewett TH, et al. Arch Virol 1977;53:287–94.
16. Fishaut M, Murphy D, Neifert M, McIntosh K, Ogra PL. J Pediatr 1981;99:186–91.
17. Holmgren J, Svennerholm A-M, Åhren C. Infect Immun 1981;33:136–41.
18. Totterdell BM, Chrystie IL, Bantavala JE. Br Med J 1980;280:828–30.
19. Welsh JK, May JT. J Pediatr 1979;94:1–9.
20. Toms GL, Gardner PS, Pullan CR, Scott M, Taylor C. J Med Virol 1980;5:351–60.
21. Zenser TV, Metzger JF. Infect Immun 1974;10:503–509.

Human Milk Banking, edited by
A. F. Williams and J. D. Baum.
Nestlé Nutrition, Vevey/Raven Press,
New York © 1984.

Effect of Heat on Specific Proteins in Human Milk

*Richard L. J. Lyster, †Manjit Hunjan, and *Eveline D. Hall

*National Institute for Research in Dairying, *Shinfield, Reading RG2 9AT, and †Hounslow TW3 4BW, England*

This work was undertaken to extend our knowledge of the heat stability of some of the proteins in human milk believed to serve protective functions in normal human infants. Although much is known about them (1,2), and some information is available on their heat stability (3–5), no extended series of measurements of the kinetics of their heat denaturation has been reported. Such a study is under way with the aim of providing the basic information needed to assess the effect of changing the time/temperature combination used in pasteurizing human milk, and some of the results are given below.

Not all the protective factors in human milk are proteins, but those that are not are either phagocytes (6), having a sensitivity to heat similar to that of *E. coli*, or heat-stable compounds such as fatty acids with antiviral activity (7).

Our studies have dealt only with proteins. Until recently it was supposed that the effect of heat on proteins was an all-or-none effect; i.e., the protein molecule was either totally denatured or unaffected. Recently, however, it has been possible to show that this is not necessarily so. Our own work on secretory immunoglobulin A (sIgA) in human milk showed that if antisera specific for different parts of the large and complex sIgA molecule were used to estimate the residual native protein after heating, then different rates of denaturation were found for different parts of the molecule.

As a result, it is not possible to use specific antisera for each protective factor to measure their rates of denaturation and assume that this has measured the loss of biological activity; instead, wherever possible, it is essential to measure the loss of biological activity directly.

In some fortunate cases, both denaturation identified by immunochemical methods and loss of biological activity can be measured fairly readily. This is the case with lactoferrin, a major whey protein in human milk that is present in particularly high concentration in colostrum (2). Lactoferrin is normally present as apolactoferrin (8), i.e., without Fe occupying the Fe-binding sites. In this form it inhibits the growth of *E. coli*, the inhibition being specifically reversed by the addition of Fe (9). Some measurements have been

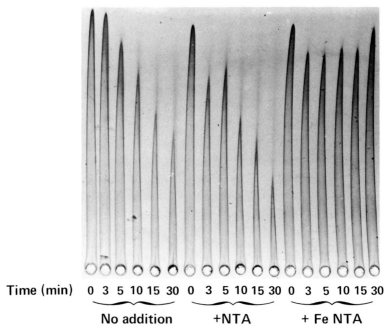

Time (min)   0 3 5 10 15 30   0 3 5 10 15 30   0 3 5 10 15 30

           No addition   **+NTA**   **+ Fe NTA**

FIG. 1. Rocket immunoelectrophoresis, using antiserum specific for lactoferrin, of milk heated at 62.5°C for various times with and without the addition of nitrilotriacetate (NTA) or the complex of NTA and Fe (FeNTA).

made of the heat stability of lactoferrin (1,4,9,10), and it has been established that it is partially denatured during pasteurization at 62.5°C for 30 min. By analogy with the similar protein ovotransferrin (11), it would be expected that the susceptibility of lactoferrin to heat denaturation would depend on whether Fe was present on the Fe-binding sites. This we have confirmed. As Fig. 1 shows, at 62.5°C, there is a steady decrease in the concentration of native apolactoferrin during an hour's heating but no significant loss of lactoferrin saturated with Fe supplied as the nitrilotriacetate (NTA) complex; as the figure shows, there is no effect of NTA on the heat denaturation of lactoferrin in the absence of Fe.

Besides using antiserum specific for lactoferrin, we have also measured the loss of its biological activity against *E. coli* using the method of Bullen et al. (9). Part of the results of a typical experiment are shown in Fig. 2. The milk sample to be tested is adjusted to pH 7.2 and inoculated with *E. coli*. The milk is then incubated

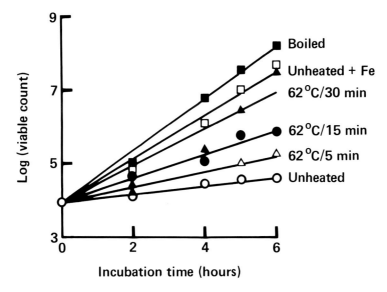

FIG. 2.   Growth of *E. coli* inoculated into human milk at pH 7.2 and incubated at 37°C after various heat treatments.

at 38°C and sampled at suitable times for plating out to obtain a figure for the viable count. Unheated samples of human milk show only a slow rate of growth; that this is because of apolactoferrin is shown by the rapid growth of *E. coli* in the two controls, one of boiled milk and one of unheated milk with Fe added. As the figure shows, heating for a short time at 62.5°C gives intermediate rates of growth.

To extract quantitative information from these results, each logarithmic growth curve was fitted to a linear expression, i.e., linear with respect to time of incubation. The slope was then expressed as a percentage of the difference between the rate of growth in boiled milk and in unheated milk. In this way, the kinetics of the loss on heating of the growth-inhibitory property of apolactoferrin were measured at several temperatures in the range 52.5°C to 62.5°C.

From these experiments it was possible to show, for example, that at 57.5°C, pasteurization of human milk would give considerably less reduction of the growth inhibition of *E. coli* than at 62.5°C.

The effect of heating to various temperatures on the survival of *E. coli* has also been measured, and the results are shown in Fig. 3. It can be seen that for any practical pasteurization process, there will be at least a log-4 reduction in viable count and usually a reduction $>$log 6. This experiment was repeated with another strain of *E. coli*, which was found to have a slightly different heat stability. These results are similar to those of Lloyd Jones et al. (12) on *E. coli, Staphylococcus aureus*, and group B β-hemolytic streptococci.

Digestibility may also be important. If pasteurization increases the digestibility of a protein, it may reduce its effectiveness in controlling the gut flora. The problem seems not to be important with lactoferrin, since Samson et al. (13) have shown that it can continue to bind Fe even after fairly extensive proteolysis. Also, we were able to show that pasteurizing at 62.5°C for 30 min had a negligible effect on the rate of proteolysis by either pepsin at pH 2 or a mixture of trypsin and chymotrypsin at pH 8. On the other hand, sIgA isolated from human milk gave different results, as shown in Fig. 4. Although pasteurization had no effect on digestion

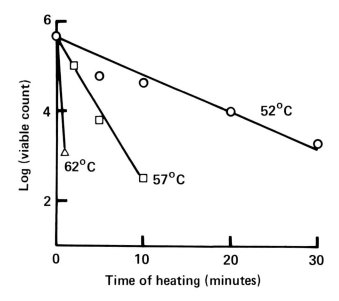

FIG. 3. Thermal death curves of *E. coli* in human milk heated at various temperatures.

by pepsin, the rate of hydrolysis by the mixture of trypsin and chymotrypsin was accelerated by pasteurization. In this experiment, purified proteins were used, and it is possible that the mixture of proteins in human milk would behave differently.

Two of the enzymes in human milk have also been studied. Alkaline phosphatase has been used for over 40 years to test for correct pasteurization of cow's milk; it is easy to test for and there is a high and fairly constant amount of it in unheated milk, and, in particular, its heat stability is just slightly greater than that of the pathogenic *Mycobacterium tuberculosis*. Unfortunately, human milk has 40 times less phosphatase than cow's milk. Nevertheless, we have measured the heat stability of the human enzyme and compared it to the bovine one, and we found no significant difference between them at any temperature in the range 50 to 70°C.

The other enzyme we have studied is the bile-salt-stimulated lipase of human milk; we have measured its heat denaturation at

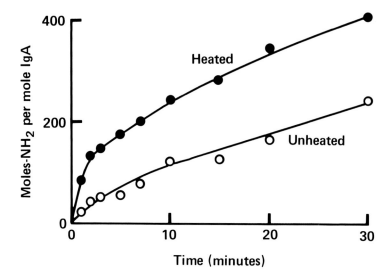

FIG. 4. Effect of heating at 62.5°C for 30 min on the rate of digestion of immunoglobulin A by a mixture of trypsin and chymotrypsin.

temperatures between 52 and 62°C. The result of measurements such as these are shown in Fig. 5. In any pasteurization process, there are three different effects of importance to consider. These are as follows:

1. *E. coli* and other organisms will be killed.
2. Some protective factors will be lost.
3. Enzymes will be denatured.

The diagram in Fig. 5 shows the effect of heating for 30 min at various temperatures. For example, at 62.5°C, the reduction in *E. coli* would be ample, alkaline phosphatase could be used to test for proper pasteurization, but lactoferrin and to some extent sIgA would be partly destroyed. On the other hand, 30 min at 57°C would give negligible loss of lactoferrin and sIgA and adequate reduction in *E. coli* count, but alkaline phosphatase would be of less use than lipase as a test enzyme. Such diagrams can now easily be constructed for

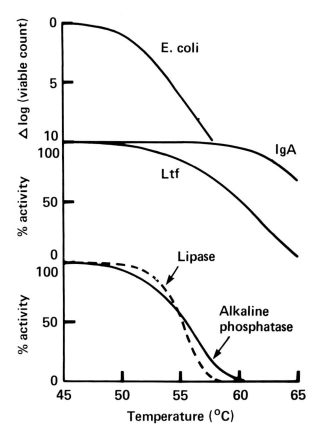

FIG. 5. Effect of heating to various temperatures for 30 min on the viable count of *E. coli (upper curve),* on lactoferrin and immunoglobulin A *(middle curves),* and on lipase and alkaline phosphatase *(lower curves).*

any desired length of heating time and should be of great assistance when one is considering any changes in the time or temperature of pasteurization of human milk.

ACKNOWLEDGMENT

This work was supported by a Project Grant from the Medical Research Council, whose assistance is gratefully acknowledged.

REFERENCES

1. Reiter B. J Dairy Res 1978;45:131–47.
2. McClelland DBL, McGrath J, Samson RR. Acta Paediatr Scand [Suppl] 1978;271:1–20.
3. Brown JD. In: Visser HKA, ed. Nutrition and metabolism of the fetus and infant. The Hague: Martinus Nijhoff, 1979:273–83.
4. Evans TJ, Ryley HC, Neale LM, Dodge JA, Lewarne VM. Arch Dis Child 1978;53:239–41.
5. Ford JE, Law BA, Marshall VM, Reiter B. J Pediatr 1977;90:29–35.
6. Paxson CL, Cress CC. J Pediatr 1979;94:61–4.
7. Welsh JK, Arsenakis M, Coelen RJ, May JT. J Infect Dis 1979;140:322–8.
8. Fransson G, Lonnerdal B. J Pediatr 1980;96:380–4.
9. Bullen JJ, Rogers HJ, Leigh L. Br Med J 1972;1:69–75.
10. Raptopouliou-Gigi M, Marwick K, McClelland DBL. Br Med J 1977;1:12–4.
11. Donovan JW, Beardslee RA, Ross KD. Biochem J 1976;153:631–9.
12. Lloyd Jones C, Jennison RF, D'Souza SW. Br Med J 1979;2:1320–2.
13. Samson RR, Mirtle C, McClelland DBL. Acta Paediatr Scand 1980;69:517–23.

Human Milk Banking, edited by
A. F. Williams and J. D. Baum.
Nestlé Nutrition, Vevey/Raven Press,
New York © 1984.

Preparation and Evaluation of Fortified Human Milk for Very-Low-Birth-Weight Infants

C. Garza, R. J. Schanler, A. S. Goldman, C. Dill, and B. L. Nichols

Children's Nutrition Research Center, Department of Pediatrics, Baylor College of Medicine, Texas Children's Hospital, Houston, Texas 77030, U.S.A.

Efforts to develop experimentally based feeding protocols using human milk for very-low-birth-weight (VLBW) infants reveal two major problems. First, there is little information on the nutrient requirements of these infants (1) and second, the description or understanding of the changes undergone by banked human milk between collection and feeding is limited (2).

We have approached the first problem by making pragmatic decisions. The range of protein and energy requirements chosen was based on the factorial calculations of Fomon et al. (3), who used intrauterine growth rates as the principal factor in their computations. Additionally, assumptions were made regarding the efficiency of nutrient utilization in the maintenance range and interindividual variation in nutrient requirements. Although such an approach does not address directly the uncertainties regarding optimal extrauterine growth rates, maturation of body composition, and development of mature metabolic abilities (4), it does provide reference points for experimental trials.

The second problem requires the determination of the composition of human milk in selected circumstances. Investigators of the Children's Nutrition Research Center, Baylor College of Medicine, Houston; in the Immunology Division of the Department of Pediatrics of the University of Texas Medical Branch, Galveston; and of the Department of Animal Science, Texas A&M University, College Station, have collaborated for 4 years in studies of the nutritional and immunologic composition of milk produced by women who delivered term (5,6) or preterm infants (7,8) and who weaned their infants gradually from the breast (9,10). We also have examined the effects of specific collection (11), storage (11,12), and processing conditions on the composition of mature human milk.

In these studies, variables such as the duration of pregnancy and lactation, completeness of emptying of the breast, time of day, diet, maternal age, and parity have been controlled. Diet and nutrient stores were controlled by qualitatively screening maternal intakes and restricting subject recruitment to middle- and upper-income groups for whom the availability of food was not a limiting factor. Central to these studies were analyses of milk of women delivering prematurely.

We have found, as have other investigators, that women delivering prematurely had levels of protein N in their milk (PM) ~21% higher than those of women delivering term infants (7). The difference in protein N between PM and milk from women delivering at term (TM) persisted for only 8 weeks and decreased with time. By the fourth week of lactation, the concentration of protein N was equal to that observed in TM at 2 weeks.

We found no differences in the caloric concentrations of these milks (7), which is in agreement with reports by Gross et al. (13), but at variance with observations made by Anderson et al. (14), who reported a 30% higher energy density in PM than TM. The gestational ages of the infants included in the Anderson study (26–33 weeks), however, were younger than in ours (30–36 weeks). Samples in the Anderson study were obtained over 24 hr; in contrast, samples in our study represented the entire content of a single breast emptied once between 8 a.m. and 12 noon. Despite these methodological differences, it appears that the disparity between our findings and those of Anderson and co-workers is caused not by higher energy concentrations in the PM assayed but by relatively lower energy values in the TM they analyzed. Our values for PM, those obtained by Gross et al., and those of Anderson et al. were 66.4, 65.4, and 68.0 kcal/dl, respectively. Analogous values from each of these laboratories for TM were 67.7, 62.3, and 58.5 kcal/dl, respectively.

From a practical standpoint, it is not uncommon for mothers to produce more milk than their VLBW infant can consume. If it were possible to identify diurnal patterns in the fat content of human milk, then one could select the most calorically concentrated milk as food for such infants. Moreover, we have found that certain key nutrients may be present in lower concentrations in PM than in TM. Mean Ca and P concentrations in PM were consistently 84 and 81%, respectively, of values obtained in samples of TM collected at 2-week intervals through the first 3 months of lactation.

In studies of milk composition during gradual weaning, we have observed that protein and Na concentrations rise as milk production falls, but other key nutrients such as Ca and energy show less consistent changes (9).

We were unable to identify a source of milk with nutrient concentrations high enough to meet the estimated needs of VLBW infants. The nutrient concentrations of the milks studied would have necessitated the feeding of volumes >175 ml/kg in order to meet our estimates of requirements. This has been a source of concern, because it is our view that a conservative regimen for the volume of fluid administered is generally appropriate for VLBW infants. Many of these infants suffer from chronic respiratory disorders, which are thought to benefit from fluid restriction. Bell et al. (15) recently reported observing a greater incidence of patent ductus arteriosus and congestive heart failure in infants managed with liberal fluid regimens. Formulas with caloric densities greater than 0.8 kcal/ml can be administered to the infant by a continuous nasogastric infusion. This is the principal feeding method used at Texas Children's Hospital and allows the delivery of higher energy and protein levels without the risks that may be entailed by high-volume feedings.

The immunologic composition of milk has been more difficult to determine. We have measured the concentrations of lysozyme, lactoferrin, secretory IgA (sIgA), total IgA, sIgA antibodies to a pool of *E. coli* antigens, and leukocytes in TM through 2 years of unrestricted lactation (5,6). Lysozyme levels fell transiently during the first 4 weeks and then rose dramatically over the next 20 weeks. Lysozyme levels remained stable thereafter for 2 years. Lactoferrin levels fell over the first 12 weeks and then remained stable for the remainder of the 2-year period we have studied. The IgA, both total and secretory, fell over the first 12 weeks and then rose over the next few weeks to levels observed at 4 weeks and remained at this level thereafter. Leukocyte levels fell over the initial 4 weeks and remained low for the duration of the period studied. During weaning, levels of these components either rose modestly or remained stable.

The pattern of compositional changes for certain immunologic factors differed substantially between PM and TM (8). Lysozyme and lactoferrin levels were greater in PM during each 2-week interval of the 3 months of observation. As in TM, sIgA is the predominant form of IgA in PM. Both total IgA and sIgA were observed to rise linearly between the sixth and 12th week of lactation. Leukocyte concentrations were of particular interest, and we found that viable leukocyte numbers in PM were lower at 2 weeks and higher at 12 weeks than in TM. Whether or not these differences are beneficial to the premature infant is not clear, nor are the mechanisms responsible for these differences apparent. Nevertheless, there are differences between PM and TM, and there is an obvious need to establish the *in vivo* functions of these components as well as the intakes necessary to ensure that they are effective.

Evaluations of collection, storage, and processing protocols were conducted either before or simultaneously with the studies that have been described. These were performed to define banking procedures to be used in the feeding protocol. Initial studies compared the composition of milks obtained by hand expression or gentle suction applied by an electric pump (11). Differences in volume and concentrations of fat suggested that the electric pump provided more representative samples, especially from mothers inexperienced with hand expression.

The effects of storage in Pyrex®, polyethylene, and polypropylene containers at 4°C also were evaluated (11). The concentrations of immunologic factors listed above and of Cu, Zn, Na, Fe, vitamin A, and protein N were measured at 4 and 24 hr of storage. Nutrient concentrations were not affected to a measurable extent by these treatments. The concentrations of several immunologic factors, however, were affected, but the changes were not related to the container used for storage with two exceptions (11). Concentrations of sIgA antibodies to *E. coli* antigens fell much more in milks stored in polyethylene containers. Also, after 24 hr, more macrophages, neutrophils, and lymphocytes were measured in the fluid phase of milks stored in Pyrex than in samples stored in polypropylene, although neither container was clearly better. Polypropylene containers, however, were chosen for all subsequent studies because there were significant losses of sIgA antibodies in polyethylene bags, there was difficulty in handling the flexible bags, and Pyrex containers were easily broken.

The effects of storage at 37, 4, and $-72°C$ in polypropylene containers have also been evaluated (11). Ascorbic acid showed the most marked changes with storage of the nutrients studied. Its concentration in milk stored at 4°C for 24 hr was 60% of the value observed after 4 hr storage at the same temperature. At 48 hr, the concentration fell to ~40% of the 4-hr value. Values were comparable in milks stored at 4 hr at 4 and 37°C and for 24 hr at $-72°C$. The transient maintenance of ascorbic acid concentrations suggests that it is protected, at least temporarily, by other factors that are oxidized more easily or that it is compartmentalized in such a way that it is protected. The decrease in ascorbic acid levels with prolonged storage suggests that other labile components might be oxidized too.

Generally, noncellular immunologic factors were highest in samples stored at 37°C regardless of storage time. Notable exceptions were total IgA and sIgA, for which similar values were observed regardless of the storage temperature. Lymphocytes, on the other hand, were present in highest numbers in samples stored at 4°C, but ³H-thymidine incorporation following PHA stimulation decreased progressively with time at all storage temperatures.

These studies indicate that many constituents are preserved when banked human milk is stored at 4°C for periods of 24 hr or less. Although some immunologic components appeared to be preserved better at 37°C, concomitant studies of bacterial growth indicated that there were many problems in preventing bacterial overgrowth when milk was maintained at this temperature.

THE PREPARATION OF HUMAN MILK FRACTIONS

The next series of experiments focused on the preparation of skim and cream fractions that could be added easily to PM and thereby increase its protein and energy densities. Levels were achieved that would permit the use of preparations for feeding VLBW infants containing ~450 mg N/kg and ~130 kcal/kg while the intake volume was maintained at ~130 ml/kg for the first 3 to 4 weeks and 160 ml/kg for the remaining 3 to 4 weeks of study. Our first choice was to use human milk components (Fig. 1) to obtain the skim and cream fractions. A short-time/high-temperature protocol was evaluated to process donor milk (DM) for this purpose. Heating DM at 72°C for 15 sec had only slight adverse effects on potentially heat-labile nutrients and preserved the immunologic identity of the proteins studied (IgA, lactoferrin, and lysozyme) at acceptable levels. This treatment also had adequate bactericidal effects and could be shown to destroy added cytomegalic virus.

For the preparation of skim and cream fractions, donor milk was screened to minimize the use of milk possibly contaminated with pathogens and pollutants. Acceptable milk was heated as described above in an APV heat exchanger with heating and cooling times of less than 5 sec. Cream and skim fractions were prepared from the heat processed DM by using a DeLaval cream separator. The cream fraction was lyophilized and stored at −20°C in foil-laminated pouches. The skim fraction was dialyzed to reduce the lactose

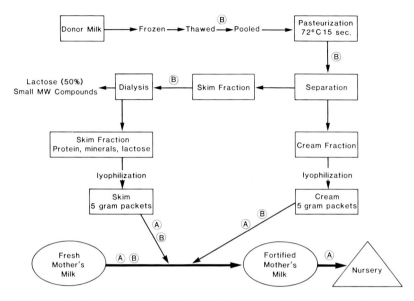

FIG. 1. Outline of protocol followed in the preparation of skim and cream fractions from donor milk: *(A)* laboratory analysis; *(B)* bacteriology.

content by ~50% against a solution containing Ca, K, Na, P, Mg, Cu, Mn, and Fe salts that was made up to maintain the mineral-to-N ratio in the skim milk. The end product of this process was lyophilized and stored, as was the cream fraction. These fractions are used to fortify PM to levels (− 346 mg N/dl and 100 kcal/dl) that meet conservative fluid requirements or to lower levels when more liberal fluid intakes are indicated.

Milk from mothers of premature infants was analyzed periodically to determine its total N and caloric density. Analyzed fractions of skim and cream were added to this milk in the proportions necessary to provide the infant with the desired levels of N and energy. Eventually, our goal was to compare clinical outcomes between infants fed this type of human milk preparation and those fed synthetic formula in isonitrogenous and isocaloric amounts. The design should permit us to test the *in vivo* significance of the functional components of human milk. Before this comparison

TABLE 1. *Description of VLBW infants fed fortified banked human milk*

Parameter	First period	Second period
n	10	7
Birth weight (g)	1,191 ± 183	1,207 ± 114
Gestational age (weeks)	29.0 ± 0.7	30.0 ± 0.5
Age during balance (days)	17.0 ± 4.0	33.0 ± 3.0
Weight gain (g/kg/day)	16.0 ± 5.0	18.0 ± 5.0

could be carried out, however, it was important to assess the utilization of N and fat from the human milk preparation described.

These assessments were conducted in a series of metabolic studies. Very-low-birth-weight infants of mothers who were planning to breast feed were enrolled from the neonatal nurseries of Texas Children's Hospital, Houston. The infants had to be 28 to 30 weeks gestation, approximate weight for gestational age at birth, and free of prolonged respiratory difficulties and major congenital anomalies. It also was required that they be on full enteral feeds by 15 days of life. The breast-feeding consultant met with the mother and family of the infant to review the protocol, which described the initiation, establishment, and maintenance of lactation without a suckling infant. Instructions were given for the collection and daily delivery of the mother's milk to the hospital. There, the milk from each mother was fortified with individually determined amounts of lyophilized fractions of skim and cream. The milk was usually fed within 24 hr of collection and seldom after 36 hr. Two feeding periods were evaluated. Human milk was fortified to a caloric density of 1.0 kcal/ml and was fed at ~130 ml/kg per day via a continuous nasogastric infusion for the first month. The second 4-week period entailed the use of milk fortified to ~0.8 kcal/ml and fed at 160 ml/kg per day. Ninety-six-hour balance studies were conducted during each period as part of the total assessment of the feeding protocol. Table 1 summarizes selected subject parameters, and Table 2 outlines their intakes. For both periods, N from processed DM accounted for ~28% of the total N fed. This was not the case for fat. In the first period, ~37% of the total fat fed came from processed DM, and 14% in the second period.

The utilization of N from PM and processed DM was compared by regression of the amount of N absorbed versus the amounts of N from PM and DM that were fed. This calculation was performed to assess the apparent digestibility of N from these two sources. In both balance periods, N from DM and PM was highly digestible. The regression coefficients calculated from the data of the first balance were 0.99 for DM and 0.90 for PM. In the second balance period, the analogous values were 0.95 and 1.00, respectively. Each of these coefficients was significant at $p<0.05$. The utilization of proteins was also evaluated by regression of the amount of N retained versus the amounts of N from DM and PM that were fed. The regression coefficients for DM and PM N in the first balance period were 0.80 and 0.80, respectively ($p<0.05$). In the second period, the values were considerably lower, 0.43 and 0.61, respectively. However, only the coefficient for PM was significant.

We have speculated about causes of possible differences in the coefficients by estimating the efficiency with which N was retained in both periods. The lower values in the second balance period may reflect a trend toward efficiencies seen in older children and adults who are consuming maintenance levels of protein (16). Efficiencies close to 65% are reported for these groups. Conversely, the high

TABLE 2. *Intake of VLBW fed fortified banked human milk*

	First period	Second period
N (mg/kg)	469.0 ± 51.0	468.0 ± 46.0
N from PM (mg/kg)	338.0 ± 58.0	340.0 ± 55.0
N from DM (mg/kg)	131.0 ± 32.0	128.0 ± 48.0
Fat intake (g/kg)	7.3 ± 0.7	6.8 ± 0.8
Fat from PM (g/kg)	4.6 ± 0.7	5.8 ± 0.5
Fat from DM (g/kg)	2.7 ± 0.6	1.0 ± 0.6
Gross energy (kcal/kg)	136.0 ± 5.0	136.0 ± 5.0

values observed in the first balance period may reflect a failure to meet the requirement for protein; in that case, a higher efficiency might be expected. Alternatively, the lower values in the second balance period may reflect a progressive deficit of a nutrient or nutrients that limited the efficiency of N utilization. The results of one additional analysis should be noted here. The regression of nitrogen retention versus the amounts of nitrogen absorbed and metabolizable energy was also calculated. In the first balance, we observed a mean increase of 2.1 mg N per added kilocalorie; in the second balance, this value dropped to 1.0 mg N per added kilocalorie. Although it is too early to comment on the statistical significance of these differences, it is of interest to make comparisons with analogous values obtained from studies in adults. Earlier work done in adults indicates an improvement in nitrogen retention of 2 to 4 mg per added kilocalorie when N and energy are provided at the maintenance range and no other nutrients are limiting (17). The apparent decrease from 2 to 1 mg N per added kilocalorie suggests that energy or another nutrient may limit the efficient utilization of N. These are speculations that require completion of the study before more definite statements can be made. However, the available data suggest that N from both sources is used equally.

We assessed the bioavailability of fat in a similar manner. The quantity of fat that was absorbed was regressed against the quantities of fat from PM and DM that were fed. In the first balance, fat from both sources was absorbed to a similar extent. The coefficients relating fat absorption to the levels of fat intake from DM and PM were 1 for both sources. These results suggest that fat from both sources was absorbed very efficiently.

We anticipate completion of these studies in the next few months. If preliminary findings are confirmed, that nitrogen and fat from processed and fresh milk are absorbed and retained with similar efficiencies, comparisons with data from similar experiments in infants fed synthetic formulas will be particularly useful. The use of fresh PM fortified with skim and cream fractions permits isonitrogenous and isocaloric feeding studies that evaluate the efficacy of human milk in promoting optimal nutrient utilization and immune function.

ACKNOWLEDGMENTS

The publication of this work is supported by a contract from the NICHD, DHHS #1-HD-8-2-28, and USDA/ARS, Children's Nutrition Research Center, Department of Pediatrics, Baylor College of Medicine and Texas Children's Hospital. The authors gratefully acknowledge the editorial review by E. R. Klein.

REFERENCES

1. American Academy of Pediatrics, Committee on Nutrition. Pediatrics 1977;60:519–30.
2. Fomon, SJ. Am J Public Health 1977;67:361–3.
3. Fomon SJ, Ziegler EE, Vasquez HD. Am J Dis Child 1977;131:463–7.
4. Heird WC. Am J Dis Child 1977;131:468–9.
5. Goldman AS, Garza C, Nichols BL, Goldblum R. J Pediatr 1982;100:563–7.
6. Goldman AS, Garza C, Goldblum RM. Acta Paediatr Scand 1983;72:461–462.
7. Garza C, Johnson CA, Butte NF, Smith EO, Nichols BL. Pediatr Res 1981;15:532.
8. Goldman AS, Garza C, Nichols BL, Johnson CA, Smith EO, Goldblum RM. J Pediatr 1982;101:901–5.
9. Garza C, Johnson CA, Smith EO, Nichols BL. Am J Clin Nutr 1983;37:61–65.
10. Goldman AS, Garza C, Goldblum RM. Acta Paediatr Scand 1983;72:133–134.
11. Garza C, Johnson CA, Harrist R, Nichols BL. Early Hum Dev 1982;6:295–303.
12. Goldblum RM, Garza C, Johnson CA, Nichols BL, Goldman AS. Nutr Res 1982;1:449–59.
13. Gross SJ, David RM, Bauman L, Tomarelli RM. J Pediatr 1980;96:641–4.
14. Anderson GH, Atkinson SA, Bryan MH. Am J Clin Nutr 1981;34:258–65.
15. Bell EF, Warburton D, Stonestrut BS, Oh W. N Engl J Med 1980;302:598–603.
16. Irwin MI, Hegsted DM. J Nutr 1981;101:385–430.
17. Garza C, Scrimshaw NS, Young VR. Am J Clin Nutr 1976;29:280–7.

Human Milk Banking, edited by
A. F. Williams and J. D. Baum.
Nestlé Nutrition, Vevey/Raven Press,
New York © 1984.

Effects of Different Heat Treatments on Some Human Milk Constituents

*V. Barrois-Larouze, †S. Jorieux, *S. Aubry,
**L. Grimonprez, and †G. Spik

*Lactarium de Paris, Paris, France; **Laboratoire de Biochimie, Faculté de Pharmacie de Montpellier, Montpellier, France; and †Laboratoire de Chimie Biologique, Université des Sciences et Techniques de Lille I, 59655 Villeneuve d'Ascq Cédex, France

The 17 milk banks in France collect about 90,000 liters of milk per year (1). Since 1947, the heat treatment employed has been tyndalization (65°C for 20 min carried out three times) in accordance with the 1954 Department of Health Report (2). An up-to-date (1983) report reviewing the installation and working requirements in milk banks is at present being prepared.

This study was carried out to test equipment for pasteurizing human milk and also to measure the effect of heat treatment on some of the major milk constituents. Several papers have been published on this topic (3,4); the present study was carried out using commercial equipment currently available on the market.

MATERIALS AND METHODS

Milk samples were obtained from 20 to 40 mothers who donated their milk to the Paris Milk Bank (Lactarium). In most instances the milk was collected using an electric pump (Egnell) or a manual pump. The milk was frozen or kept at +4°C for no more than 48 hr before being collected from the mother's home. The samples were pooled in 4-liter batches. The milk used in each machine and cycle was obtained from different pools. The milk samples used for biochemical studies were frozen at the milk bank before and after pasteurization and kept frozen until tested.

Holder Pasteurization Equipment

Holder pasteurization equipment comprised three machines that were lent to the Paris Lactarium. In all our experiments with the Holder pasteurizers, one bottle filled with milk was placed in the center of the bath, and the others were filled with water. The characteristics of each machine are as follows (Tables 1 and 2):

The Oxford Human Milk Pasteurizer

The bath temperature is 63°C, and milk is maintained at that temperature for 30 min. The milk containers are plastic and hold 100 ml. The total milk volume per cycle is 4 liters, and each cycle takes 100 min.

The CM80 Pasteurizer

The bath temperature is also maintained at 63°C for 30 min; 7.2 liters in 200-ml glass baby bottles can be pasteurized at one time, and the cycle takes 120 min. A feature of this machine is that the bottles are gently shaken during the cycle.

The Lyon Pasteurizer

Because technical assistance was available, it was possible to change the bath temperature easily. We used three different procedures: 65°C for 30 min and 58°C for 30 min done once or twice. The same milk bottles as for the CM80 were used (volume 200 ml). The total volume per cycle is 9.6 liters. The duration of a cycle is 120 min.

Tyndalizer

The *Tyndalizer* is a somewhat old-fashioned machine and is still used in milk banks in France. The milk is heated at ~65°C for 20 min three times at 24-hr intervals.

Thonon High-Temperature Short-Time Pasteurizer

The milk flows into a tube and is maintained at 70°C for 14 to 17 sec depending on the output, which is between 28 and 33 liters per hour. The temperature is reduced to 4°C in 30 to 45 sec.

BACTERIOLOGICAL TESTS

Bacteriological tests were carried out in the Paris Lactarium according to the procedures described in Table 2. At least 15 studies were performed for each type of equipment at each given temperature.

Protein Assay Techniques

Fractions enriched in secretory immunoglobulin A (sIgA), lactotransferrin, and lysozyme were prepared from thawed defatted milk. The latter was decaseinated and then fractionated using a concentration gradient of $(NH_4)_2SO_4$ and a pH gradient as described by Montreuil et al. (5). The sIgA was isolated from fraction P_4 under conditions described by Pierce-Cretel et al. (6). Lactotransferrin was purified from fraction P_{7-8} by ion-exchange chromatog-

TABLE 1. *Equipment and procedures*

Equipment	Heating Temperature (°C)	Duration (min)	Milk volume per container (ml)	Total milk volume per cycle (liters)
Oxford Human Milk Pasteurizer	63	30	100	4.0
CM80	63	30	200	7.2
Lyon Human Milk Pasteurizer	58	30	200	9.6
	65	30		
Human Milk Tyndalizer	65	20	200	20.0
Thonon HTST Pasteurizer[a]	70	14–17 sec[b]	Continuous flow	28–33 liters/hr

[a]High-temperature, short-time pasteurization.
[b]Cooling to 4°C, 30–45 sec.

TABLE 2. *Bacteriological tests*

Before pasteurization
  1. Blood agar medium (total mesophilic flora); 0.1 ml of milk diluted
     1/1,000 and 1/10,000
  2. Chapman medium *(Staphylococcus)*; 0.1 ml of milk diluted 1/10
  3. Drigalsky medium (enterobacteria); 0.1 ml of milk diluted 1/100
After pasteurization
  Blood agar medium (total mesophilic flora); 0.1 ml of undiluted milk

---

raphy according to the procedure described by Spik et al. (7). Lysozyme was obtained from fraction P_{7-8} by ion-exchange and gel-filtration chromatography. Monospecific antisera to sIgA, lactotransferrin, and lysozyme were produced in rabbits according to the procedure of Vaitukatis et al. (8).

Levels of sIgA and lactotransferrin were determined by the radial immunodiffusion technique of Mancini et al. (9).

The iron-binding capacity of lactotransferrin was determined after saturating defatted milk with sufficient $FeCl_3$ in citrate/bicarbonate pH 8.6 reagent (10). Free iron was removed by ion-exchange chromatography, and the protein precipitated in acid conditions. The iron released from the lactotransferrin was measured using sulfobathophenanthrolin reagent (11).

Lysozyme activity was assayed using the enzymatic lysoplate, which measures the lysozyme-mediated degradation of heat-killed *Micrococcus lysodeikticus* cells (12).

Carbohydrate Assay Techniques

After thawing at room temperature, the milk samples were defatted by centrifuging at $+4°C$. Ten milliliters of each sample was dialyzed overnight at $+4°C$ against 100 ml of distilled water. All dialyzable fractions were lyophilized and analyzed by electrophoresis and chromatography (13,14). For electrophoresis, 10 mg of each fraction was placed on the anode side of No. 3 Whatman filter paper. Electrophoresis was carried out over 15 hr at 7 V/cm using a water–acetic pyridine–acid buffer at pH 5.4, and spots were stained using aniline oxalate reagent at 105°C.

For chromatography, 4 mg of each fraction was put on No. 3 Whatman paper and 4 mg on No. 3 MM Whatman paper. Chromatography was performed for 15 and 36 hr, respectively, using a solution of pyridine:ethyl acetate:distilled water (1:2:2). Spots were stained by the same procedure used after electrophoresis.

RESULTS

Bacteriology

The total mesophilic colony count before pasteurization varied considerably (10,000 to 10,000,000 CFU/ml). Our criterion for adequate pasteurization was that the total mesophilic flora should be < 10 CFU/ml. This criterion was met using all the procedures with the exception of the 58°C/30 min method with the Lyon Human Milk Pasteurizer; however, after a second treatment at the same temperature, the total mesophilic count was < 10 CFU/ml with this machine.

Changes in Milk Constituents

Table 3 shows the modifications of sIgA, lactotransferrin, iron-binding capacity, and lysozyme activity after pasteurization. Several experiments were done with each type of equipment and procedure. Table 3 shows the mean results. The values after pasteurization are expressed as a percentage of the initial values. In view of the small number of studies, care should be exerted in making comparisons, and we consider our results as preliminary.

Good results were obtained with the Oxford Human Milk Pasteurizer at 63°C for 30 min, but only three experiments were done. Considerable variations were observed using the same procedure (63°C for 30 min) or similar (65°C for 30 min) with different types of equipment. The first results obtained with the Lyon Human Milk Pasteurizer (58°C for 30 min repeated twice) were particularly encouraging. The results of the Thonon High-Temperature Short-Time continuous-flow pasteurizer were also satisfactory.

TABLE 3. *Protein survival after pasteurization*

| Equipment | No. of studies | Heating | | IgA (% survival) | Lactotransferrin (% survival) | Iron-binding capacity (% initial value) | Lysozyme (% initial activity) |
		Temp. (°C)	Duration (min)				
Oxford Human Milk Pasteurizer	3	63	30	87.1	61.6	78.3	ND
CM 80/6	8[b]	63	30	71.1	17.3	4.8	95.8
Lyon Human Milk Pasteurizer		58	30	92.7	89.3	ND[a]	ND
	2[c]	58	30	99.2	100.0	94.3	96.9
	3	65	30	56.8	15.8	ND	92.4
Human Milk Tyndalizer	3	65	20	75.2	28.1	45.5	ND
Thonon HTST Pasteurizer	3	70	15 sec	81.3	39.0	55.3	ND

[a]ND, no data.
[b]One cycle.
[c]Two cycles.

No modification of acid oligosaccharides, monocarbohydrates (galactose, glucose, fucose, *N*-acetylglucosamine, *N*-acetylneuraminic acid) and polysaccharides (tri-, tetra-, penta-, and hexasaccharides) was observed with any of the methods used.

DISCUSSION

The aim of heat treatment is to kill bacteria with the minimum loss of milk constituents. All the equipment and procedures proposed by the manufacturers produced efficient bacterial killing. We therefore tried to lower the heating temperature to 58°C for 30 min but obtained poor bacteriological results. Effective pasteurization was, however, obtained by repeating the cycle twice.

The results obtained with the Oxford Human Milk Pasteurizer at 63°C for 30 min confirmed the results of others using the same equipment and the results of experiments carried out previously at the same temperature (3,4,16). Immunoglobulin A seems to be preserved better than lactotransferrin and iron-binding capacity. This is confirmed by the results obtained with the CM80 and the Lyon Human Milk Pasteurizer. Our data confirm the stability of lysozyme previously observed by Ford (3) and Eyers (15).

Discrepancies in results obtained with the 63°C/30 min method suggest that factors other than time and temperature should be taken into account. In particular, it should be noted that only the Lyon Human Milk Pasteurizer records milk temperature during Holder pasteurization. In other types of equipment, only the bath temperature is measured. We carried out further studies to investigate this point. Results obtained with the Lyon Human Milk Pasteurizer using the same milk show that the type of milk container (glass or plastic) does not seem to be important. Similarly, exposure to heat for 20 min instead of 30 min is not associated with better biochemical preservation. Among other factors, the volume of each milk container and shaking might modify the thermokinetics. Another factor that might modify the protein survival is the pH. At 58°C for 30 min with the Lyon Human Milk Pasteurizer, the destruction of IgA and lactotransferrin tends to decrease as the pH increases.

Depending on the daily quantity of milk dealt with by a milk bank, we propose the following recommendations:

1. A milk bank that collects more than 6,000 liters a year could use the High-Temperature Short-Time Pasteurizer by which 30 to 40 liters can be pasteurized per hour with a good protein preservation. Precautions should be taken to avoid bacterial contamination when filling bottles after pasteurization.

2. A milk bank that collects $<$6,000 liters/year could pasteurize batches of 7 to 10 liters at a time at a given temperature in 200-ml bottles. As a bacteriological test is done to check the heat treatment after each cycle, it would be best to try to pasteurize at a temperature as low as possible (17). If the result is unsatisfactory, we suggest pasteurizing twice, because at 56 or 58°C, the loss of IgA and lactotransferrin is less after two exposures at these temperatures than after one exposure at temperatures $>$60°C. With a 200-ml container, 60°C seems to be a critical temperature above which proteins are damaged.

3. Similar considerations apply to milk banks that receive only small amounts of milk daily; small containers (100 ml) should be used so that the milk is heated and cooled quickly.

ACKNOWLEDGMENT

This work was supported by a grant from the French Ministry of Health.

REFERENCES

1. Barrois V, Junot M, Larouze B. Ann Pediatr 1982;29:489–93.
2. Journal Officiel de la République Française. 1954;27 Aug:8327.
3. Ford J. J Pediatr 1977;90:29–35.
4. Raptopoulou-Gigi M. Br Med J 1977;1:12–14.
5. Montreuil J, Chosson A, Havez R, Mullet S. CR Soc Biol 1960;154:732.
6. Pierce-Cretel A, Pamblanco M, Strecker G, Montreuil J, Spik G. Eur J Biochem 1981;114:169–78.
7. Spik G, Strecker G, Fournet B et al. Eur J Biochem 1982;121:413–9.
8. Vaitukatis J, Robbins JB, Nieschlag E, Ross GT. J Clin Endocrinol 1971;33:988–91.
9. Mancini G, Carbonara AO, Heremans JF. Immunochemistry 1965;2:235–54.

10. Azari P, Baugh RE. Arch Biochem Biophys 1967;118:138–44.
11. Société Française de Biologie Clinique. Ann Biol Clin 1977;35:275.
12. Osserman EF, Lawlor DP. J Exp Med 1966;124:921–51.
13. Grimonprez L, Montreuil J. Biochimie 1975;57:695–701.
14. Kobata A, Yamashita K, Tashibana Y. Methods Enzymol 1978;50:216–20.
15. Eyres R, Eliott R, Howie R, Farmer K. NZ Med J 1978;87:134–5.
16. Liebhaber M. J Pediatr 1977;91:897–900.
17. Wiss M, Han V, Harris D, Baum J. Early Hum Dev 1982;7:71–81.

Human Milk Banking, edited by
A. F. Williams and J. D. Baum.
Nestlé Nutrition, Vevey/Raven Press,
New York © 1984.

Loss of Immune Components During the Processing of Human Milk

S. Freier and J. Faber

Department of Pediatrics, Shaare Zedek Hospital, Jerusalem 91002, Israel

Although milk banks have been in existence for more than 50 years (1), the past decade has seen a resurgence of interest in their functions and systems of operation. In spite of this, there is as yet no consensus as to how breast milk should be processed and stored. Some milk banks prefer to freeze milk (2) to preserve, as far as possible, the immune factors present. Others insist on carefully controlled Holder pasteurization (3), forfeiting some of the immune factors but destroying the majority of potential pathogens (2). In view of the current controversies, we would like to review some of the salient facts as they have been reported so far. Our objective is to scrutinize the relevant data, which will enable us to define the optimal method of processing milk.

THE PATHOGENS

It is uncommon for breast milk to be sterile (4,5). The bacteria present in breast milk include those that can be regarded as harmless commensals, such as coagulase-negative *Staphylococcus* and *Streptococcus viridans*, as well as "potential" pathogens (Table 1). These so called "potential" pathogens have, however, only rarely been implicated as causes of neonatal morbidity. There are reports of two nursery outbreaks of *Salmonella kottbus* infection (7,8), one of *Salmonella typhimurium*, and one of *E. coli*, in which human milk was believed to be the source of infection (2,9). In two of these

123

TABLE 1. *The prevalence of bacteria in raw breast milk (%)*

	Method of collection		
Presence of bacteria	Water, sterile swab, electric pump (ref. 9)	Drip milk (ref. 4)	Manual under supervision (ref. 6)
Sterile	0	3	65.2
Commensals			
Coagulase-negative *Staphylococcus*; *Streptococcus viridans*	78	82	22
Potential pathogens Coagulase-positive *Staphylococcus*; enterobacteria; group A and B *Streptococcus*	22	15	12.8
Total:	100	100	100

outbreaks the milk was heat processed. These observations, therefore, do not resolve the case for or against pasteurization.

It is noted in Table 1 that one group of investigators claimed that 65% of specimens were sterile (6). It is obviously of great importance to establish whether this is the result of personal hygiene and aseptic technique or whether the bacteriological methods employed were less sensitive than those of other investigators. Other studies show that the bacterial flora of breast milk are largely derived from the skin and areola of the breast (5). Additional clinical trials are required within individual units to compare different methods of breast cleansing and milk collecting.

A more elusive threat is that posed by viruses. Herpes viruses including cytomegalovirus (CMV) as well as rubella virus and hepatitis B surface antigen (HBsAg) have been demonstrated in breast milk (10–13). In the case of hepatitis B, there is evidence that the presence of surface antigen in breast milk does not produce a carrier state in the infants of HBsAg carrier mothers (14). Thus, when infants of carrier mothers become infected, infection is not through the breast milk. These observations, however, concern babies fed on the breast and not babies fed donor milk. Uncertainty also exists about CMV. Some 10 to 17% of women excrete CMV in their milk (15), and there is epidemiological evidence linking viral excretion in milk with infant acquisition of CMV during the first year of life (13). In these infants, virus was excreted in urine and saliva for several years, but no untoward clinical effects were noted. An additional factor to consider is that infants born to CMV-seropositive mothers have natural protection in the form of IgG antibodies. Such protection is absent in the blood of infants born to seronegative mothers. Caution must therefore be exercised in giving milk from CMV-seropositive mothers to seronegative infants. However, to date, there are no convincing descriptions of morbidity in full-term newborns as a result of breast-milk-acquired CMV.

THE IMMUNE FACTORS

Cellular Factors and Specific Antibodies

The most numerous cells in human milk are the macrophages. Their concentration in breast milk rapidly diminishes after birth and by 6 weeks is 1/100 that at 2 weeks (16). This large and metabolically active phagocyte is capable of synthesizing many of the antibacterial substances present in breast milk, including complement components C_3 and C_4, lysozyme, and lactoferrin (17). In addition, macrophages seem to exert a helper function on IgA-producing plasma cells *in vitro*; in the presence of macrophages, more IgA is released and for longer periods. The phagocytic function of macrophages and neutrophils has been shown to be directed against *Staphylococcus, E. coli*, and *C. albicans* (18). Oral moniliasis, being easy to detect, might be a useful marker in comparing clinical effects of raw and pasteurized milk.

T and B lymphocytes are present in breast milk in the same relative proportions as in blood. Functionally, however, breast milk lymphocytes respond to mitogens in a manner different from that of blood lymphocytes (19). Moreover, it is believed that particular clones of lymphocytes accumulate in breast tissue. B lymphocytes in breast milk actively secrete immunoglobulins, mainly IgA, although immunoglobulins G, M, E, and D are also present in small quantities. The total amount of IgA imbibed by the infant remains at the considerable level of 1 g/day throughout lactation. The fate of ingested IgA is unknown. There are several possibilities. In rabbits it has been shown that the neonatal intestine possesses specific receptors for breast milk secretory IgA (20). It remains to be determined whether a similar phenomenon exists in the human infant. Another possibility is that IgA becomes adsorbed onto the mucus overlying the glycocalyx, as is the case in the adult intestine (21). In either case, IgA would be anchored for prolonged periods to the wall of the intestine, where it could serve to prevent bacterial adhesion, promote bacterial agglutination, neutralize viruses, and complex food proteins.

The repertoire of specific antibodies in breast milk is considerable and varies from mother to mother. It is determined to some extent by the bacterial, viral, and food antigens present in the mother's gastrointestinal and respiratory tracts (22,23). Sensitized lymphocytes from intestinal and bronchial-associated lymphoid tissues migrate to breast tissue and there secrete the appropriate antibodies. Antibodies have been described against enteroviruses, rotavirus, herpes simplex, CMV, influenza, arboviruses, rubella, and respiratory syncitial virus (11). One would also like to know whether specific antibodies to hepatitis B virus exist in breast milk of mothers secreting the virus. The presence of such antibodies would be of great theoretical and practical interest and could influence decisions on the best way of processing breast milk.

Cellular immunity, presumably conferred by breast milk T cells, has been studied to only a limited extent. It has been shown that tuberculin-reactive T cells in breast milk can confer this reactivity to the infant's peripheral blood lymphocytes, but only for a brief period (24). How this transfer of cellular immunity from mother's milk to the infant's peripheral blood is achieved is another area for future research.

Nonspecific Humoral Factors

Unsaturated lactoferrin is effective against *E. coli* and *C. albicans* (25). Its concentration shows a gradual decline during lactation (26). Lysozyme, which is active against *E. coli* and *Salmonella*, shows a threefold rise. The lactoperoxidase system is active against *Streptococcus*, *Pseudomonas*, *E. coli*, and *S. typhimurium*. However, salivary peroxidase activity in the newborn is greater than milk lactoperoxidase, suggesting that the salivary activity represents the more important antibacterial agent (27). All nine components of complement have been detected in breast milk (28). Their function, if any, is a matter of conjecture, as the main intestinal immunoglobulin, IgA, is not complement dependent. Other humoral factors of antibacterial and antiviral potential are chemotactic factors, bifidus factor, lipid-associated staphylococcal resistance factors, monoglycerides with antiviral activity, α_1-antitrypsin, and other protease inhibitors (11). In addition, a variety of immunoregulatory substances, including macrophage migratory inhibition factor, IgA-stimulating factors, interferon, and T-cell immunosuppressive substances, have been identified in human colostrum and milk (11).

Control of Viral Infection

In addition to specific viral antibodies belonging largely to IgA, various nonspecific factors may help to curb viral infections. Certain free fatty acids and monoglycerides have the capacity to attack the envelopes of some viruses (29). Other nonlipid fractions, which so far have eluded identification, have been shown to be active against vesicular stomatitis virus (30), herpes simplex virus (31), and rotavirus, one of the most common causes of infantile gastroenteritis (30). Free interferon has not been detected in human milk, but milk lymphocytes can be stimulated to produce it. Whether such stimulation does in fact take place is still unknown (32).

FACTORS ADVERSELY AFFECTING THE ANTIINFECTIVE PROPERTIES OF BREAST MILK

Some of the antiinfective properties of human milk may be partly or wholly destroyed during processing. Relevant factors include the type of container used for storing milk, the length of storage, and the effects of cooling to 4°C, of freezing, and of heating.

The Effect of the Container

Goldblum and co-workers (16) have shown that storage of mature milk at 4°C for 24 hr in polypropylene containers caused a significant decrease in lysozyme and lactoferrin, whereas polyethylene containers dramatically reduced the titer of secretory IgA antibodies to *E. coli* somatic antigens without decreasing the concentration of total or secretory IgA. Moreover, there was a significant decrease in the functional capacity of the cellular components irrespective of which container was employed. An additional interesting finding that arose out of these investigations was the fact that colostrum appeared to impart greater stability to its components than did mature milk. None of the cellular or humoral immunological factors investigated was diminished when colostrum was stored at 4°C for 24 hr in any of the containers mentioned.

Effect of Heat

Not surprisingly, milk leukocytes survive best when incubated at near body temperature. Heating milk to 56°C will drastically reduce (33), and Holder pasteurization at 62.5°C for 30 min will completely eliminate (34), all cellular elements in breast milk.

Both pasteurization and lyophilization cause marked reductions of IgG and IgM. Pasteurization at 62.5°C will reduce the concentration of IgA by 33%, and the minute amounts of IgE present in raw breast milk will disappear altogether. Together with the reduction of total IgA, there is a drop in antibodies to *E. coli* (34). Similarly, the amount of lactoferrin is affected by pasteurization, but lysozyme is stable. In view of the many antibacterial and antiviral factors present in breast milk, one cannot draw conclusions from the fact that some factors are destroyed by heating and that others are stable. More meaningful information can be obtained by comparing the total antibacterial activity of raw and pasteurized breast milk. Studies of this type show that the antibacterial activity may be seriously impaired by pasteurization (35). No similar observations exist on antiviral activity, but as the antiviral factors are more resistant to heat, it is likely that this activity is better preserved on pasteurization.

The Effect of Freezing

Freezing has less effect on the immune components of human milk, particularly if the changes in temperature take place rapidly. Reynolds et al. (36) describe a method of collecting and rapidly freezing breast milk using the breast pump devised by Yamanouchi and Igarashi (37). The advantages of this pump are simplicity and ease of sterilization. From the pump, the milk is transferred to plastic bags designed by the same investigators. These bags are robust and withstand freezing and thawing. If relatively small bags are used, the milk can be frozen rapidly. The authors examined each specimen of milk in the raw state, after storage at − 20°C overnight, and after 1 and 4 weeks. Each specimen was examined for bacterial contamination, bacteriostatic activity, cellular and immunological components, fat, and amino acids. The results showed that there was no appreciable rise in bacterial counts on storage, and bacteriostatic activity was preserved for at least 1 week. A surprisingly large number of cells survived freezing and storage.

CONCLUSIONS

The present divergence of opinion on milk processing results largely from the lack of decisive clinical trials comparing pasteurized with raw milk. In these circumstances, our views are based largely on inference from *in vitro* observations colored by personal bias. In this chapter, we have reviewed some of the extensive literature on the immune properties of breast milk. However, none of the data presented can obviate the need for clinical trials to settle current controversies. One interesting recent clinical study suggested that raw colostrum or breast milk could reduce the prevalence of infections among neonates even when used as a supplement to formula feeds (6). This important study unfortunately did not examine the use of pasteurized human milk.

In the future, therefore, we must endeavor to answer a number of questions; we would like to define only a few that arise from our study:

1. Can the present methods of collection of breast milk be improved in order to obtain a greater number of sterile specimens?
2. Apart from the four reported outbreaks of infection *(Salmonella* and *E. coli)* in which faulty technique was to blame, is there any evidence in properly organized milk banks that bacteria in raw breast milk cause morbidity?
3. Does the presence of HBsAg reflect the existence of HB virus in breast milk? Could this be ascertained by a search for core antigen (HBcAg) or "e" antigen (HBeAg) or the specific DNA polymerase?
4. What is the fate of breast milk IgA in the human intestine?
5. Do ingested intact monocytes and macrophages from breast milk have any role in the infant's immune regulation?
6. What is the morbidity in two comparable groups of infants treated in the same unit receiving Holder pasteurized milk and rapidly frozen raw milk?

The answers to these questions will not be obtained easily; careful attention to study design and analysis will be vital, but only by objective clinical studies will agreement on the optimal method for milk processing be reached.

ACKNOWLEDGMENT

We should like to thank the Miriam Fish-Coven Fund for financial assistance.

REFERENCES

1. Siimes MA, Hallman N. J Pediatr 1978;94:173–4.
2. Bjorksten B, Burman LG, de Chateau P, Frederikzon B, Gothefors L, Hernell O. Br Med J 1980;281:765–9.

3. Baum JD. In: Freier S, Eidelman AI, eds. Human milk: its biological and social value. Amsterdam: Excerpta Medica, 1980:179–86.
4. Carrol L, Osman M, Davies DP, McNeish AS. Lancet 1979;2:732–3.
5. Eidelman AI, Szilagyi G. Obstet Gynaecol 1979;53:550–2.
6. Narayanan I, Prakash K, Prabhakar AK, Gujral VV. Acta Paediatr Scand 1982;71:441–5.
7. Center for Disease Control. Morbid Mortal Week Rep 1971;20:154.
8. Ryder RW, Crosby-Ritchie A, McDonough B, Hall WC III. JAMA 1977;238:1533–4.
9. Silver HG, Albritton WL, Clark J, Friesen P, White FMM. Can J Publ Health 1977;68:479–82.
10. Dunkle LM, Schmidt RR, O'Connor DM. J Pediatr 1979;63:250–1.
11. Ogra PL, Fishaut M, Theodore C. In: Freier S, Eidelman AI, eds. Human milk: its biological and social value. Amsterdam: Excerpta Medica, 1980:115–21.
12. Shiraki K, Yoshihara N, Kawana T, Yasui H, Sakurai M. Am J Dis Child 1977;131:644–7.
13. Stagno S, Reynolds DW, Pass RF, Aford CA. N Engl J Med 1980;302:1073–6.
14. Boxall EH, Derso A, Flewett TH. In: Freier S, Eidelman AI, eds. Human milk: its biological and social value. Amsterdam: Excerpta Medica, 1980:159–63.
15. Dworsky M, Stagno S, Pass RF, Cassady G, Alford C. J Pediatr 1982;101:440–3.
16. Goldblum RM, Goldman AS, Garza C, Johnson CA, Nichols BL. Acta Paediatr Scand 1982;71:143–4.
17. Goldman AS, Smith CW. J Pediatr 1973;82:1082–90.
18. Lawton JWM, Shortridge KF. Lancet 1977;1:253.
19. Diaz-Jouanen E, Williams RC. Clin Immunol Immunopathol 1974;3:248–50.
20. Nagura H, Nakane PK, Brown WR. J Immunol 1978;120:1333–9.
21. Walker WA, Isselbacher KJ. N Engl J Med 1977;297:767–73.
22. Fishaut M, Murphy D, Neifert M, McIntosh K, Ogra PL. J Pediatr 1981;99:186–91.
23. Tomasi TB, Larson L, Challacombe S, McNabb P. J Allergy Clin Immunol 1980;65:12–9.
24. Schlesinger JJ, Covelli HD. Lancet 1977;2:529–32.
25. Kirkpatrick CH, Green I, Rich RR, Schade AL. J Infect Dis 1972;124:539–44.
26. Goldman AS, Garza C, Nichols BL, Goldblum RM. J Pediatr 1982;100:563–7.
27. Gothefors L, Marklund S. Infect Immun 1975;11:1210–5.
28. Michael JC, Ringenback R, Hottenstein S. J Infect Dis 1972;124:445–8.
29. Welsh JK, Skurrie IJ, May JT. Infect Immun 1978;19:395–8.
30. Matthews THJ, Nair CDG, Lawrence MK, Tyrell DAJ. Lancet 1976;2:1387–9.

31. Sabin AB, Fieldsteel AH. Pediatrics 1962;29:105–8.
32. Emodi G, Just M. Scand J Immunol 1974;3:157–60.
33. Paxson CL, Cress CC. J Pediat 1979;94:61–3.
34. Sunshine P, Asquith MT, Liebhaber M. In: Freier S, Eidelman AI, eds. Human milk: its biological and social value. Amsterdam: Excerpta Medica, 1980:178–90.
35. Roberts SA, Severn M. Br Med J 1978;277:1196.
36. Reynolds GJ, Meade HJ, Brown BJ, Fitzgerald TS, Isherwood IM, Lewis Jones DI. Br Med J 1982;284:560.
37. Yamanouchi I, Igarashi I. In: Freier S, Eidelman AI, eds. Human milk: its biological and social value. Amsterdam: Excerpta Medica, 1980:191–6.

Human Milk Banking, edited by
A. F. Williams and J. D. Baum.
Nestlé Nutrition, Vevey/Raven Press,
New York © 1984.

Characterization and Biological Role of Human Lactotransferrin Complexes

*Geneviève Spik, *Sylvie Jorieux, *Joël Mazurier,
**Jean Navarro, †Charles Romond, and *Jean Montreuil

*Laboratoire de Chimie Biologique et Laboratoire Associé au CNRS 217,
Université des Sciences et Techniques de Lille I, 59655 Villeneuve d'Ascq Cédex,
France; **Hôpital Bretonneau, Pavillon Legroux, 75018 Paris, France; and
†Faculté de Pharmacie, Laboratoire de Microbiologie, 59045
Lille Cédex, France

Several epidemiologic studies have indicated that breast feeding protects infants from bacterial and viral infections and from allergy (1–6). Recent prospective studies performed by Chandra (7) in an industrialized country and in a developing one confirm that in both countries, breast-fed infants have lower morbidity than those artificially fed. One of the most striking differences between breast- and bottle-fed infants concerns the fecal pH and bacterial flora. The feces of breast-fed infants contain predominantly *Bifidobacterium bifidum*, whereas those of bottle-fed infants are characterized by the presence of high quantities of *Bacteroides, Clostridium*, and *Escherichia coli* (8). According to Beerens et al. (9), cow's milk as well as sheep's milk, pig's milk, and artificial human milks do not promote the growth of *Bifidobacterium bifidum* but do show activity on *Bifidobacterium infantis* and *Bifidobacterium longum*.

Human milk therefore contains two kinds of factors that contribute to the intestinal protection. The first group consists of antibacterial components such as secretory immunoglobulin A (sIgA), lactotransferrin (also called lactoferrin), lysozyme, and lactoperoxidase. The second group includes *Bifidobacterium bifidum* growth-promoting factors, which are essentially oligosaccharides. The nature of the antibacterial and growth-promoting factors has been summarized in several review articles (10–17). Comparative study of the biochemical compositions of human and bovine milk (18,19) has shown that the essential constituents considered as protecting the infant's intestinal tract are absent or are present in low concentration in cow's milk.

Several procedures have been applied for isolating the oligosaccharides (20) and proteins (18,21,22) from human milk. In the course of experiments with electrophoretic separation, differences were noticed in the mobility of lactotransferrin present in milk and that of lactotransferrin extracted from this milk. The differences may be explained by the interaction of lactotransferrin with proteins and with nonprotein compounds present in the milk. Since it has not been determined whether the complexed lactotransferrin possesses biological properties similar to purified lactotransferrin, we have attempted to isolate the lactotransferrin complexes and to analyze their bacterial activities. Fractionation of milk proteins was performed by precipitation with ammonium sulfate, and the bacteriostatic activity as well as the *Bifidobacterium bifidum* growth-promoting activity of the different fractions were determined *in vitro*. Subsequently, the fraction possessing the highest antibacterial activity was selected for the treatment of infants with acute diarrhea.

The present report concerns the characterization of lactotransferrin–lysozyme and lactotransferrin–glycopeptide complexes in human milk and the description of the bacteriostatic activities of these complexes *in vitro* and *in vivo*.

MATERIALS AND METHODS

Isolation of the Milk Fractions

Samples of human milk were collected from a local milk bank, pooled, and frozen at $-20°C$ until use. The thawed milk was defatted by centrifugation and then decaseinated. The whey proteins were fractionated by a combined concentration gradient of $(NH_4)_2SO_4$ and pH gradient as described by Montreuil et al. (23) and Montreuil

(18). The lactotransferrin–lysozyme complex was isolated by ion-exchange chromatography on SP-Sephadex column and by gel filtration on an Ultrogel ACA-44 column.

Identification and Estimation of the Proteins

The proteins were submitted to electrophoresis on cellulose polyacetate strips using a barbital sodium buffer, pH 8.6. The lactotransferrin complexes were identified by cross immunoelectrophoresis using a monospecific antiserum to lactotransferrin according to the procedure described by Weeke (24).

The estimation of lactotransferrin was determined by a single radial immunodiffusion technique (25). Lysozyme activity was assessed from the enzymatic lysoplate assay, which quantitates the lysozyme-mediated lysis of killed *Micrococcus lysodeikticus* cells (26).

Bacterial Activities

Antibacterial activities were analyzed by measuring the inhibition of growth of *Escherichia coli* $O_{111}B_4$ in a Ringer–tryptone medium (27) containing the different milk fractions. The optical density was followed using an automatic biophotometer.

The test for bifidus growth factors was performed by the method described by Neut et al. (28) using *Bifidobacterium* strains freshly isolated from infant feces. The antibacteriostatic activity of the milk fraction P_{7-8} was tested on five infants suffering from acute diarrhea. These infants were fed on a regimen containing 2 g of the P_{7-8} fraction over a period of 8 days. The intestinal flora of these infants was determined before and after treatment.

RESULTS

Analysis of the Milk Fractions

A total of seven whey precipitates was isolated after fractionation of human milk proteins with ammonium sulfate. The nature of the proteins of each precipitate was identified by electrophoresis and by immunoelectrophoresis (Table 1).

Bacterial Activities of the Milk Fractions

The bacteriostatic activity of the different fractions as well as the capacity of these fractions to promote the growth of *Bifidobacterium bifidum*, *Bifidobacterium longum*, and *Bifidobacterium infantis* are given in Table 2. These results show that the most interesting fraction is the precipitate P_{7-8}, which contains *Bifidobacterium* growth-promoting factors and possesses bacteriostatic activity.

Analysis of the Fraction P_{7-8}

The estimation of different proteins by the radial immunodiffusion method has shown that fraction P_{7-8} contains 70% lactotransferrin, 6% secretory component, and 7% lysozyme. In addition, this fraction contains 17% carbohydrates as shown by chemical

TABLE 1. *Composition of the precipitates obtained by fractionation of human milk whey with ammonium sulfate (29)*

Fraction	$(NH_4)_2SO_4$ saturation	pH	Nature of the proteins
P_1	0.33	7.0	Galactothermin; sIgA; α-lactalbumin; secretory component
P_2	0.33	4.6	α-Lactalbumin; sIgA; serum albumin; secretory component; lactotransferrin; $α_1$-antitrypsin (traces)
P_3	0.33	3.8	Serum albumin; α-lactalbumin; lactotransferrin (traces)
P_4	0.50	7.0	sIgA; IgG; IgM; lactotransferrin (traces)
P_{5-6}	0.50	3.8	Serum albumin; lactotransferrin; sIgA; α-lactalbumin
P_{7-8}	0.75	4.6	Lactotransferrin; secretory component; sIgA; lysozyme; serum albumin (traces)
P_9	0.75	3.8	Glycopeptides; peptides; lactotransferrin; $α_1$-antitrypsin; lysozyme
P_{10}	1.0	3.8	Peptides; glycopeptides; $α_1$-antitrypsin (traces)

TABLE 2. *Bacterial activities of the different fractions obtained from human milk whey by ammonium sulfate fractionation*

Bacterial activity	Fraction								Dialyzable oligosaccharides
	P_1	P_2	P_3	P_4	P_{5-6}	P_{7-8}	P_9	P_{10}	
Inhibition of the growth of *Escherichia coli* $O_{11}B_4$	−	+	−	+	+	+ +	−	−	−
Bifidobacteria									
Bifidobacterium bifidum	−	−	−	−	−	+	−	−	+ +
Bifidobacterium longum	−	−	−	+	+	+ +	−	−	−
Bifidobacterium infantis	−	−	−	+	+	+ +	−	−	−

analysis. Cross immunoelectrophoresis of the fraction P_{7-8} in the presence of a rabbit serum antihuman lactotransferrin shows that the profile is quite different from those obtained from a sample of purified lactotransferrin or from fractions P_{5-6} and P_9. In particular, two different types of lactotransferrin may be identified in this fraction (Fig. 1).

Isolation and Properties of the Lactotransferrin–Lysozyme Complex

In order to identify the lactotransferrin complexes present in fraction P_{7-8}, the latter was submitted to ion-exchange chromatography on an SP-Sephadex column. A fraction containing lactotransferrin and lysozyme was separated from the other components of P_{7-8}. This fraction was further submitted to gel filtration on an Ultrogel AcA-44 column, and free lysozyme was separated from a lactotransferrin–lysozyme complex. The complex has a molecular weight of 110,000 and results from the stoichiometric association of 2 moles of lysozyme per mole of lactotransferrin. As shown in Fig. 2, the electrophoretic mobility of the lactotransferrin–lysozyme

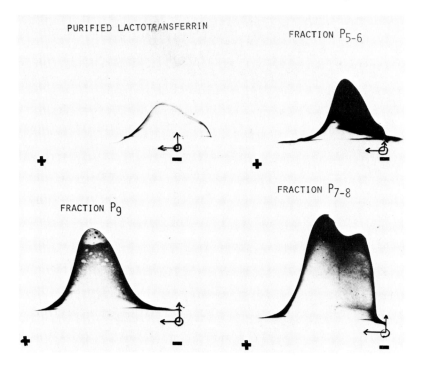

FIG. 1.   Crossed immunoelectrophoresis in the presence of a rabbit serum antihuman lactotransferrin of purified lactotransferrin and of fractions P_{5-6}, P_{7-8}, and P_9 obtained by fractionation of human milk whey.

complex was quite different from those of pure lactotransferrin and of pure lysozyme. The difference in the electrophoretic mobilities explains the presence of two peaks in the profile of P_{7-8} characterized by cross immunoelectrophoresis.

Characterization of Lactotransferrin–Glycopeptide Complexes

Addition of increasing amounts of precipitate P_{10} containing essentially glycopeptides having a molecular weight of 20,000 to pure lactotransferrin leads to the formation of complexes between lactotransferrin and glycopeptides having an electrophoretic mobility more anodic than that of pure lactotransferrin (Fig. 3) (29,21).

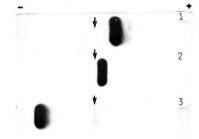

FIG. 2. Polyacetate electrophoresis of lactotransferrin–lysozyme complex (1), purified human lactotransferrin (2), and purified human lysozyme (3). *Arrows* indicate the starting points.

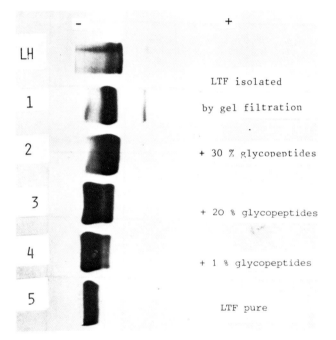

FIG. 3. Electrophoretic mobility of pure lactotransferrin (LTF) compared to lactotransferrin complexes obtained by adding increasing amounts of the glycopeptides present in fraction P_{10} to pure lactotransferrin.

Such complexes probably exist in the fraction P_{7-8} but have not been isolated. Indeed, a dissociation occurs during ion-exchange chromatography on SP-Sephadex as a result of the weakness of the ionic associations of the lactotransferrin–glycopeptides complex.

Biological Role of P_{7-8} Fraction

In vitro, the fraction P_{7-8} appears to be more bacteriostatic than pure lactotransferrin. Therefore, we have employed this fraction for the treatment of five babies suffering from acute diarrhea and intolerance to bovine milk protein. The babies received 2 g of P_{7-8} for a period of 8 days, and the effect of this diet was assessed by identifying the duodenal microflora. Results did not show a decrease of the number of enteropathogenic strains such as *Escherichia coli* or *Streptococcus*; however, a significant decrease was noted in the case of *Staphylococcus*, *Pseudomonas maltophilia*, and *Erwinia*. Subsequent to treatment, the tolerance of the children toward the bovine and human milk proteins was restored.

DISCUSSION

Lactotransferrin, by its iron-binding capacity, represents one of the most powerful bacteriostatic constituents of human milk. Its activity is retained in the gut as a result of its resistance to digestive proteases. In fact, we have demonstrated (30) that lactotransferrin is still present in the feces of breast-fed infants and that it has retained its ability to bind ferric ions reversibly. We have shown in this chapter that in human milk, lactotransferrin interacts with other constituents such as lysozyme and glycopeptides. We believe that the interaction of lactotransferrin with these constituents increases the biological activity of the lactotransferrin. In a recent publication, Perraudin and Prieels (31) have shown that the protoplasts produced by the action of lysozyme on *Micrococcus luteus* are agglutinated by free human and bovine lactotransferrins. Thus, lysis and agglutination appear to be increased by the presence of lactotransferrin–lysozyme complex.

It is generally agreed that the first step of infection is mediated by bacterial adherence to mucosal surfaces. This interaction is explained by a mechanism that involves recognition of sugars by specific bacterial lectins (32). In experiments carried out in collaboration with Dr. Mirelman (33,34), an inhibition of *Shigella flexneri* binding to the mucus extracted from colonic cells of guinea pigs was observed in the presence of free fucose and of asialoglycopeptides containing fucose residues. The glycopeptides that form complexes with lactotransferrin are fucose-rich. Therefore, the lactotransferrin, which contains two glycans with fucose residues, and the complexes of lactotran ferrin with fucose-rich glycopeptides may constitute powerful po ntial inhibitors for the adhesion of some bacteria.

These results represent strong arguments in favor of the use of therapeutic milks supplemented with lactotransferrin and with polysaccharides containing monosaccharide units such as mannose, which are able to inhibit the adhesion of bacteria, *Escherichia coli* in particular (35), to the mucosal surface.

In summary, the importance of fresh human colostrum and milk for the prevention of *E. coli* diarrhea (36,37) may result from the presence of several milk constituents, among which are sIgA, lactotransferrin, lysozyme, and glycopeptides. Human lactotransferrin possesses a bacteriostatic activity applicable by a ferriprivation mechanism. In addition, it has been shown *in vitro* that lactotransferrin and sIgA together have a powerful bacteriostatic effect against pathogenic strains of *Escherichia coli* responsible for diarrhea that is greater than their effect when used alone (38–40). An increase in the effect of lactotransferrin is also demonstrable *in vitro* by complex formation among this protein and lysozyme and sugars. However further experiments *in vivo* are necessary in order to assess the clinical significance of this observation.

ACKNOWLEDGMENTS

This work was supported in part by the C.N.R.S. (Laboratoire Associé 217) and by the Ministère de la Santé. We are indebted to the Lactariums of Lille and Paris for providing human milk and to J. P. Decottignies for his skillful technical assistance.

REFERENCES

1. Robinson M. Lancet 1951;210:788–92.
2. Math LH, Urrutia JJ, Gordon JE. Trop Geogr Med 1967;19:247–51.
3. Larsen SA, Homer DR. J Pediatr 1978;92:417–8.

4. Cunningham AS. J Pediatr 1979;95:685–9.
5. Ellestad-Sayed J, Coodin FJ, Dilling LA, Haworth JC. Can Med Assoc 1979;120:295–8.
6. Fallot ME, Boyd JL, Oski FA. Pediatrics 1980;65:1121–4.
7. Chandra RK. Acta Paediatr Scand 1979;68:691–4.
8. Bullen CL, Willis AT. Br Med J 1971;3:338–43.
9. Beerens H, Romond C, Neut C. Am J Clin Nutr 1980;33:2434–9.
10. György P. In: Wolstenholme EW, O'Connor M, eds. Nutrition and infection. Boston: Little, Brown, 1967:59–65.
11. Mata LJ, Wyatt RG. Am J Clin Nutr 1971;24:976–81.
12. Hanson LA, Winberg J. Arch Dis Child 1972;47:845–50.
13. Brown RE. Am J Clin Nutr 1973;26:556–61.
14. Goldman AS, Smith CW. J Pediatr 1974;82:1082–7.
15. Gerrard JW. Pediatrics 1974;54:757–9.
16. Reiter B. Ann Rech Vet 1978;9:205–24.
17. Welsh JK, May JK. J Pediatr 1979;94:1–9.
18. Montreuil J. Ann Nutr Aliment 1971;25:A1–A37.
19. Blanc B. In: Bourne GH, ed. World review of nutrition and dietetics, vol 36. Basel: S Karger, 1981:1–89.
20. Grimmonprez L. Ann Nutr Aliment 1971;25:A39–A79.
21. Spik G. Ann Nutr Aliment 1971;25:A81–A134.
22. Bezkorovainy A, Nichols JH. Pediatr Res 1976;10:1–5.
23. Montreuil J, Chosson A, Havez R, Mullet S. CR Acad Sci [D] (Paris) 1960;154:732–6.
24. Weeke B. In: Axelsen NH, Krøll J, Weeke B, eds. A manual of quantitative immunoelectrophoresis. Oslo: Universitetsforlaget, 1973:47–56.
25. Mancini, G, Carbonara AO, Heremans JF. Immunochemistry 1965;2:235–54.
26. Selsted ME, Martinez RJ. Anal Biochem 1980;109:67–70.
27. Reiter B, Brock JH, Steel ED. Immunology 1975;28:83–95.
28. Neut C, Romond C, Beerens H. Reprod Nutr Dev 1980;20:1679–84.
29. Descamps J. [Thesis]. Lille: University of Lille, 1974.
30. Spik G, Brunet B, Mazurier-Dehaine C, Fontaine G, Montreuil J. Acta Paediatr Scand 1982;71:979–85.
31. Perraudin JP, Prieels JP. Biochim Biophys Acta 1982;718:42–8.
32. Sharon N, Eshdat Y, Silverblatt FJ, Ofek I, eds. Ciba conferences on adhesion and microorganism pathogenicity. London: Pitnam Press, 1980.
33. Izhar M, Nuchamowitz Y, Mirelman D. Infect Immun 1982;35:1110–18.
34. Pierce-Crétel A, Strecker G, Montreuil J, et al. In: Proceedings of the 7th international symposium on glycoconjugates (in press).
35. Eshdat Y, Ofek I, Yashouv-Gan Y, Sharon N, Mirelman D. Biochem Biophys Res Commun 1978;85:1551–9.
36. Larguia AM, Urman J, Stoliar OA, et al. Environ Child Health 1977;289–90.

37. Barlow B, Santulli TV, Heird WC, Pitt J, Blanc WA, Schullinger JN. J Pediatr Surg 1974;9:587–95.
38. Bullen JJ, Rogers HJ, Leigh L. Br Med J 1972;8:69–75.
39. Spik G, Chéron A, Montreuil J, Dolby JM. Immunology 1978;35:663–71.
40. Stephens S, Dolby JM, Montreuil J, Spik G. Immunology 1980;41:597–603.

Human Milk Banking, edited by
A. F. Williams and J. D. Baum.
Nestlé Nutrition, Vevey/Raven Press,
New York © 1984.

Practical Problems in Conducting Comparative Trials of Feeding Regimens in Very-Low-Birth-Weight Infants

A. F. Williams

The University Department of Paediatrics, John Radcliffe Hospital, Oxford OX3 9DU, England

It has been suggested that the growth of very-low-birth-weight infants fed human milk may be restricted by protein (1) and energy deficiency. If this is the case, it is logical to suppose that enrichment of human milk with human milk proteins and fats will accelerate their growth. It is tempting to suppose that this hypothesis could be proven simply and objectively by a clinical trial. An account of the practical problems encountered in testing this hypothesis in clinical practice is given here. We conclude that there are many obstacles to relating gross nutrient intake and growth differences between very-low-birth-weight infants by clinical trial methods. These factors include difficulty in measuring growth and nutrient intake with accuracy and large variations in morbidity between and within infants.

POOLED HUMAN MILK AND THE VERY-LOW-BIRTH-WEIGHT INFANT—THE PROBLEM

Most of the controversy over the suitability of human milk for feeding the very-low-birth-weight infant relates to pooled human milk collected by human milk banks. Human milk is considered by some to be too low in nutrient concentration (1) to provide sufficient substrate for the very-low-birth-weight infant to achieve fetal growth rates. However, cross-sectional standards of birth weight at various gestational ages may not represent patterns of longitudinal growth for individual infants born prematurely, and the clinical sequelae of growth rates below those seen in the fetus have not been characterized. There is therefore room for caution in stating that human milk is quantitatively deficient in nutrients, and when nutrient quality is considered, there is strong *in vitro* evidence to suggest that the constituents of human milk are more appropriate than those of artificial formulas. Many of the proteins can be shown to possess biological functions, potentially conferring specific and nonspecific immunity and digestive functions (e.g., bile-salt-stimulated human milk lipase) on the infant. These systems are elaborate, and it is attractive to propose that the very-low-birth-weight infant fed pooled human milk will be clinically advantaged, but clear direct proof as shown from clinical trials is, in most cases, lacking.

Most clinical studies have compared groups of infants fed human milk with groups fed artificial formulas. These are beset with methodological problems. First, it is difficult to achieve true random allocation of infants—in many studies, the group of infants fed artificial milk has been the group whose mothers did not wish to breast feed. Second, numbers have usually been small. Third, clinical staff know, as do the experimenters, to which group the patient belongs; the effects of staff attitudes on perinatal clinical trials have been remarked on previously (2), and these may be equally important in feeding studies.

Thus, the problem is not simple. Many questions require experimental testing. Clinicians must decide the relative importance of each question according to their practice, as this factor affects the outcome measure that is chosen. One might ask "Does pooled human milk protect the infant from infection?" The outcome measure would be the incidence of proven infection; however, measurement of a significant protective effect would require a large study in the special-care nurseries of industrialized societies, where antibiotics are used in abundance. By contrast, Naryanan (3) has demonstrated such effects in a nursery in India.

In developed countries, the question of most concern is "Is the growth of very-low-birth-weight infants fed pooled human milk restricted by nutritional deficiency?" This is the question that is discussed here. How easily can it be objectively answered by a clinical trial?

The Hypothesis

If the growth of very-low-birth-weight infants is restricted by nutritional deficiencies in pooled human milk, it is logical to suppose that enrichment of pooled human milk will accelerate growth. Consideration of the protein content of human milk and the maturity of biochemical pathways in the very-low-birth-weight infant (4) suggests that supplementary human milk proteins will be well tolerated. The hypothesis to be tested, therefore, is that enrichment of pooled human milk with human milk proteins and human milk fats will accelerate the growth of preterm infants without a metabolic cost.

The Contribution of "Lactoengineering" to the Study

The term "lactoengineering" has been employed by Baum generally to describe methods of altering human milk composition. This is methodologically a valuable tool because it allows controlled preparation of human milks of widely differing composition, allowing blind comparisons of enriched human milk and pooled human milk to be made for the first time.

The Method of "Lactoengineering"

For the study considered here, the purpose of lactoengineering was simply to provide a human milk substantially enriched in composition in comparison with pooled human milk supplied by the human milk bank. In the case of the John Radcliffe Hospital Milk Bank, "drip" breast milk (DBM) is collected. The composition, collection, and processing of this milk are described elsewhere (5). Composition was altered by first skimming fat from a 4-liter batch of milk (centrifugation at 1,500 g, 4°C, 20 min). Skimmed milk was then concentrated fourfold by ultrafiltration using an Asahi Medical AM10 "hollow-fiber" dialysis cartridge (95% molecular weight cutoff 6×10^4).[1] The skimmed milk concentrate prepared in this way was lyophilized to a powder. Powder and fat from each 4-liter batch was then resuspended in another 4-liter batch of human milk. This preparation was described as a "human milk formula" (HMF). It was pasteurized and microbiologically screened before use.

The protein and energy composition of the experimental "human milk formula" and the control "drip" breast milk are shown in Table 1. Energy content was determined by bomb calorimetry (16) of triplicate lyophilized samples. Protein content was determined by the Biuret technique (7).

The Design of the Controlled Clinical Trial of "Human Milk Formula"

The study was a randomized blind comparison of enriched human milk with unaltered pooled human milk. Random allocation of very-low-birth-weight infants to feeding groups is, in practice, difficult because many mothers elect to begin expressing milk to feed their own infants. Exclusion of these infants would be selective, and in any case, experience shows that these infants, in later weeks, often require an additional source of milk as part or the whole of their dietary requirement.

In this study, infants receiving any enteral feeds at 7 days of age were randomly allocated, using random-number tables, to a control

TABLE 1. *Composition of the feeds*

	Drip breast milk	Human milk formula
Protein (g/100 ml)	1.2 ± 0.13	1.91 ± 0.37
Gross energy (kcal/100 ml)	57 ± 3	81 ± 16

[1]Manufacturer's information. Supplied by Kimal Scientific Products Limited, Uxbridge, U.K.

group or an experimental group without regard to the mother's own milk supply. The control group received pooled human milk from the milk bank when mother's own milk was insufficient to meet the fluid demands of the infant or was unavailable; the experimental group received "human milk formula" according to the same clinical indications. Mothers were not told which feed their infants would receive, and consent was obtained on this understanding. It was felt that this might influence their decision to continue breast feeding. The "drip" breast milk and the "human milk formula" were supplied in containers of identical appearance so that the clinical staff, parents, and anthropometrists were unaware which feed a baby was receiving. Twenty consecutive inborn infants with birth weight $< 1,800$ g (excluding small-for-date infants) were identified for inclusion in the study. Two sets of parents refused consent, so that 18 infants were studied. All feeds were administered by orogastric tube, the volume of feed given was measured by syringe and recorded by the nurses. The recommended intake for each baby was 180 ml/kg/day, although in practice this was varied at the discretion of the staff. Babies were withdrawn from the trial at discharge from hospital or if clinical staff felt they were "failing to thrive."

Weight was recorded daily, or every other day, by nursing staff who used an Avery balance with resolution of ± 10 g. Length was measured weekly using a Holtain neonatal stadiometer (8), but this measurement was sometimes omitted in the sickest babies who failed to tolerate the necessary handling. Head circumference was measured using paper tapes. Measurements of length and head circumference were made in all cases by the same pair of trained observers.

In order to detect dietary protein overload in babies fed the "human milk formula," venous blood was taken once weekly from all babies, and plasma tyrosine estimated by a fluorometric method (9).

THE OUTCOME OF THE STUDY

Objective comparison of the treatment regimens was frustrated by three major considerations. First, dropout rates were considerably higher than expected; second, accurate measurements of growth over short periods were difficult; and third, a problem was created by variation in the weight trajectories of individual babies. This tended to frustrate between-group comparisons of weight gain at set postnatal ages. These aspects of the study bear separate consideration as problems for the clinical investigator.

Dropout Rates

The nursery in which this trial was carried out is a regional neonatal intensive-care referral center. None of the babies studied was outborn, but eight babies out of 18 recruited to the study were transferred to other hospitals in the region after an average stay of only 3.4 weeks (2.3–4.5 weeks). If babies transferred out were a random sample of those included, an objective comparison between the two groups would of course still have been possible. However, babies are transferred out when they are no longer sick, and at this stage, they have usually just begun to gain weight. The babies who remain are, therefore, a selected sick population, and it is likely that nutrition accounts for a much smaller proportion of the variance in growth in this group than in a group of well babies. Simple comparisons between groups receiving different gross nutritional intakes are thus reduced in their discriminatory power.

How might this problem be overcome in a trial design? Multi-center studies might be an answer in the future, provided the number of infants studied was sufficiently large to control for variations in nursery practice by randomly allocating to control and experimental groups within nurseries and not between nurseries.

The group of three babies removed by clinical staff (because of failure to thrive) deserves separate consideration. It included both of the only two babies who were totally dependent on pooled banked human milk (DBM) for their nutrition and one of the three babies totally dependent on enriched human milk (HMF) for their nutrition. Thus, although two out of the three babies totally dependent on "human milk formula" were considered to be growing adequately by clinical staff, none of the babies dependent on unenriched pooled human milk was. Because this was a blind trial, this observation may be of some interest, but the numbers are of course insufficient for any statistical comparison.

Short-Term Measurements of Growth

Weight gain is the most commonly used measure of growth in the nursery. The relative insensitivity of mechanical balances means that the most accurate measurements of weight gain are made by plotting a regression of weight against time, taking the slope of the line as weight gain in grams per day. There are two important qualifications that relate to the accuracy of this technique. First, change in weight with time in infants born preterm (unlike change in length or head circumference with time) appears to obey a power curve equation more closely than a linear regression equation (see Fig. 1). The corollary of this in making comparisons of growth rate between individuals is discussed later, but for the present, let it be assumed that the error involved in calculating weight gain over a short period of enteral feeding (e.g., 1 week) using a linear regression method is very small.

Second, the proportion of the variance in weight that is attributable to time is expressed by the square of the correlation coefficient, r^2. In a sick baby, this may be very low (see Fig. 2). In 6 out of 18 babies in the second week of life in this study, r was <0.7, but in another 6, it was >0.95. In the first case, 50% of the variance in weight can be accounted for by time, and in the second, $>90\%$ is accounted for by time. The reason for this discrepancy cannot be assumed to be attributable to differences in milk intake; it might be equally attributable to greater error in the measurement of weight in the first group. It is difficult to separate these two effects, and, hence, it is difficult to be sure that weight gain is a comparable measure of the effect of milk intake in the two groups.

When the effect of nutrition on growth is investigated in very-low-birth-weight infants, accurate short-term measurements of growth are vital because periods of enteral feeding when the baby is in a

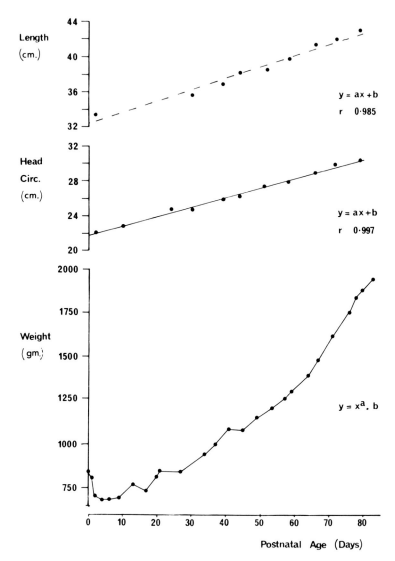

FIG. 1. Growth chart of one of the 26-week-gestation infants studied. Weight does not show a linear relationship with time, showing that weight gain interacts with postnatal age.

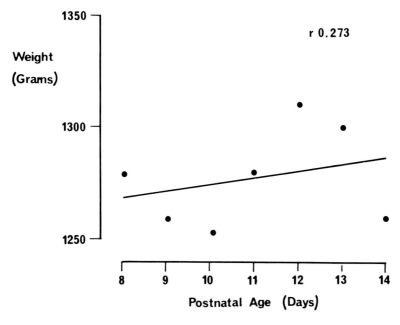

FIG. 2. Relationship of weight and time in one of the study infants during the second week of life. Large day-to-day variations in weight in sick infants can make linear regression methods unsuitable for calculation of weekly weight gain.

steady clinical state are few. They are punctuated by periods of intercurrent illness, which may involve curtailment or reduction of nutritional intake. The problem of measuring linear growth over short periods is a pragmatic one. Although measurement of crown–heel length has been shown to be a technique capable of accuracy (8), many sick babies do not tolerate the manipulation necessary to make reproducible readings. Thus, accurate measurements of crown–heel length can be difficult in the early weeks. Measurement of shorter distances (e.g., foot length) has been suggested (6) as an alternative, but there are no longitudinal studies that indicate that growth of the foot parallels growth in crown–heel length in the preterm infant. In addition, the coefficient of variation in the measurement is approximately 1.5% in our experience, and this distance is close to 33% of the weekly increment expected from the available intrauterine growth standards (10).

Comparing Rates of Weight Gain Between Individuals—The Effect of Weight Trajectories

Although we have referred to intrauterine growth as a measure of optimal postnatal growth (11) for very-low-birth-weight infants, it should be noted that so-called "intrauterine growth standards" are, more strictly, cross-sectional plots of birth weight and gestational age. It cannot be inferred that the growth trajectory of any individual infant should follow such a course. Indeed, as Brandt (12) has shown in longitudinal studies, the weight trajectory of growing preterm infants is quite different from that described by a cross-sectional plot of birth weight and gestational age.

Weight gain in growing preterm infants approximates more closely to a power curve relationship, and this is clearly seen in Fig. 1, showing the growth of an individual infant included in the study. Much variation between infants can be accounted for by the very different patterns of early weight loss over the few weeks after birth. This feature is not purely an effect of variation in nutritional intake; it can be heavily influenced by features such as severity of illness, drug therapy (e.g., diuretics), and water and electrolyte balance.

In the case of the study infants, early weight loss was very variable, even within each of the two feeding groups (Table 2). This meant that the phase of weight gain—starting at the time when infants regain birth weight—begins at very different postnatal ages.

TABLE 2. *Time taken to regain birth weight*

Group	Week 1	2	3	4	Withdrawn[a]	Discharged[a]
Control	0	1	3	2	1	1
Experimental	0	0	4	4	1	1

[a]Before regaining birth weight.

Cross-sectional comparisons of weight gain between feeding groups at set postnatal ages cannot, therefore, be made without taking into account the point that each infant has reached on his individual weight trajectory. Infants may start to gain weight at quite different postnatal ages but finish at similar points attained through different routes. Weight velocities at set postnatal ages can, therefore, be spurious. For this reason, weight gain, although a reasonable measure of nutritional state in an individual infant, has to be looked at very critically when one is making comparisons between individuals. For interindividual comparisons, measurements of linear growth velocity would not appear to be subject to these errors, since their relationship with postnatal age approximates very closely a linear regression with a constant slope at all postnatal ages (Fig. 1).

The Relationship Between Weight Gain and Gross Nutrient Intake in Individual Infants

Weight gains (g/kg/day) of the seven babies who were studied from birth to discharge are shown for each individual in Fig. 3. Each data point represents the slope of the regression of weight on

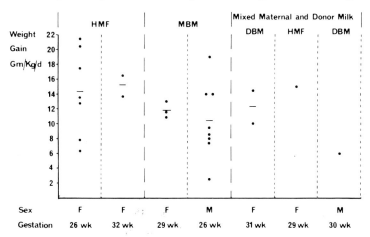

FIG. 3. Weight gains of the seven infants completing the study. Each point represents the weight gain shown during a week of pure enteral feeding. Note the large within-individual variations.

time for a 1-week period when enteral feeding was uninterrupted. This figure has been divided by the baby's average weight during the 1-week period to express weight velocity in the units shown. In the case of most babies, few weeks of uninterrupted enteral feeding were identified, explaining the paucity of data points for some individuals. Only in the case of two babies fed entirely on the "human milk formula" (HMF) could gross energy intake be stated accurately, because the energy content of the feeds had been determined by bomb calorimetry and the volume given had been measured by syringe. Although individual babies can show a wide range of weight velocities at different postnatal ages, the correlation of gross energy intake, where this was known, with weight gain was very low ($r = 0.371$, 8 df).

A study (13) examining the relationship between gross energy intake of babies fed raw expressed maternal breast milk with weight gain made similar conclusions. Several explanations may account for this. First, wide interindividual differences in nutrient absorption exist; in support of this as an explanation is the improved correlation of metabolizable energy intake with weight gain observed by others (14). Equally, energy utilization is likely to vary according to postnatal age and morbidity. Finally, in this study and in the raw expressed breast milk study referred to above (13), the range of gross energy intake provided was similar and quite high (here between 100 and 210 cal/kg/day); it is possible that energy absorption and tissue deposition are maximal at a given energy intake, making the relationship between gross energy intake and weight gain nonlinear.

Biochemistry

Two babies were found to have plasma tyrosine concentrations well outside the normal range (400 and 600 μmol/liter). These two babies belonged to a group of four infants who were dependent on human milk formula for their nutrition (one of these babies was subsequently transferred to another hospital). In one case, however, the baby had received human milk formula for only 24 hr (day 8) and had therefore not been receiving a high protein level. This prompted us to examine vitamin C intake. Normal clinical practice is to provide a multivitamin suspension (0.3 ml) from the seventh day of life. This contains 25 mg of vitamin C. Although the vitamin C content of mature expressed breast milk is quoted as 3.8 mg/100 ml (15), the vitamin C content of pooled drip breast milk was found to be lower than this in all of six pools studied (mean 1.26 mg/100 ml, range 0.8–1.9 mg/100 ml). The concentration of vitamin C in these samples fell to only 0.48 mg/100 ml (range 0.07–0.8 mg/100 ml) after pasteurization. Babies receiving pasteurized human milk, therefore, have very low intakes of vitamin C. Following this observation, subsequent babies received supplementary vitamin C (60 mg daily). No further hypertyrosinemia was seen.

CONCLUSIONS

Care was taken to design a blind randomized control trial of feeding on enriched human milk, but high dropout rates prevented statistical comparisons between groups. Other pitfalls in between-group comparisons were highlighted, which suggests that weight gain is an outcome measure subject to interaction with postnatal age and early weight loss and that where gross energy intake could be stated with confidence, it showed poor correlation with weight gain.

These findings suggest that clinical trials of feeding regimens for very-low-birth-weight infants will require large numbers of infants for study and careful choice of outcome measures. There is much current pressure to change feeding regimens, often in favor of artificial formulas, but without objective demonstration of the superiority of one regimen over another in clinical trials, these efforts should clearly be resisted.

ACKNOWLEDGMENT

This research was supported by a grant from the International Council of Infant Food Industries.

REFERENCES

1. Fomon SJ, Ziegler EE, Vazquez HD. Am J Dis Child 1977;131:463–7.
2. Silverman WA. Retrolental fibroplasia: a modern parable. New York: Grune & Stratton, 1980:140.
3. Naryanan I, Prakash K, Gujral VV. J Pediatr 1981;99:496–8.
4. Raiha N. In: Freier S, Eidelman AI, eds. Human milk: its biological and social value. Amsterdam: Excerpta Medica, 1980:15–22.
5. Gibbs JH, Fisher C, Bhattacharya S, Goddard P, Baum JD. Early Hum Dev 1977;1:227–45.
6. James DK, Dryburgh EH, Chiswick ML. Arch Dis Child 1979;54:226–30.
7. Bosset J, Blanc B, Plattner E. Anal Chim Acta 1974;70:327–39.
8. Davies DP, Holden RE. Arch Dis Child 1972;47:938–40.
9. Waalkes TP, Udenfriend S. J Lab Clin Med 1957;50:733–6.
10. Usher R, McLean F. J Pediatr 1969;74:901–10.
11. American Academy of Pediatrics. Pediatrics 1977;60:519–30.
12. Brandt I. In: Rooth G, ed. 5th European congress of perinatal medicine. Stockholm: Almqvist and Wiksell, 1976:221–9.
13. Spencer SA, Hendrickse WA, Roberton D, Hull D. Br Med J 1982;85:924–6.
14. Brooke OG, Alvear J, Arnold M. Pediatr Res 1979;13:215–20.
15. Department of Health and Social Security. In: The composition of mature human milk. Report on Health and Social Subjects 12, London: HMSO, 1977.
16. Miller DS, Payne PR. Br J Nutr 1959;13:501–8.

Human Milk Banking, edited by
A. F. Williams and J. D. Baum.
Nestlé Nutrition, Vevey/Raven Press,
New York © 1984.

Lactoengineering: A Method for the Estimation of the Human Milk Protein Requirements of Very-Low-Birth-Weight Newborn Infants

*B. S. Lindblad, *S. Hagelberg, **R. Fondén, *B. Persson, and *A. Lundsjö

*Department of Pediatrics, Karolinska Institute at St. Göran's Children's Hospital and **Arla Research and Development Department, Stockholm, Sweden*

This chapter concerns some of the observed metabolic effects of varying the protein and fat content of human milk. These modifications in the composition of human milk have been achieved without disturbing its immunological properties or lipase activity and without the addition of foreign antigen. These experiments were conducted in order to determine the nutritional requirements of very-low-birth-weight (VLBW) infants.

The hypothesis that the protein requirement is especially high during the initial period after birth in the VLBW infant is based on known fetal accretion rates (1). However, before advocating an optimal food supply, we must take into consideration the infant's metabolic tolerance to the amount given. This is particularly critical in the VLBW infant, who suffers from both limited excretion and metabolic capacity (2). Thus, in our efforts to avoid brain damage by providing sufficient energy and protein during this critical period of development, we are sailing between the Scylla of brain damage from undernutrition and the potential Charybdis of brain damage resulting from overnutrition (Fig. 1). What we need is a method of producing a "human milk formula" (3) without destroying the advantages of using human milk and yet without having to provide large volumes of water (4).

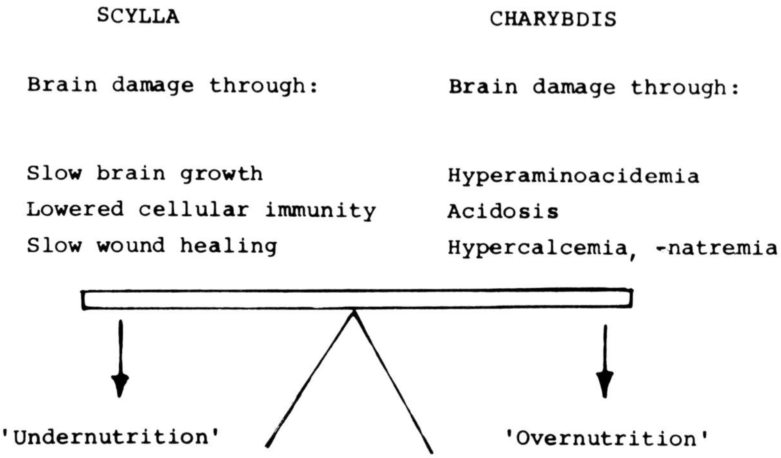

```
SCYLLA                              CHARYBDIS

Brain damage through:               Brain damage through:


Slow brain growth                   Hyperaminoacidemia
Lowered cellular immunity           Acidosis
Slow wound healing                  Hypercalcemia, -natremia
```

FIG. 1. The Scylla and Charybdis of over- and underfeeding the VLBW newborn infant.

To circumvent this problem, two different methods have been developed. In the first, the mother's own milk, or banked milk, is concentrated to provide an increased concentration of nutrients. The method potentially leads to rough handling of the immune properties of the milk and to high osmolality. The second method, which is the one we have chosen, is that of producing human milk fat and protein fractions to be added to the mother's own fresh milk or banked milk pasteurized with a special plate heat exchanger.

The homeostasis of blood amino acids is a sensitive index of protein and calorie supply in relation to requirement and to metabolic tolerance (5). We have recently reported (6) that the doubling of the human milk protein content was well tolerated by four VLBW infants given 150 to 175 ml/kg per day of their mothers' protein-fortified milk. This was evident from the acid–base balance, the free amino acid levels of whole blood, the serum urea levels, and growth, which followed the intrauterine growth curve. It has also been demonstrated that human milk supplementation prevents hypoproteinemia without causing metabolic imbalance in LBW infants fed expressed breast milk (7).

However, there are serious difficulties in defining normal levels of indices such as the free amino acid concentrations of peripheral blood in a group that should normally have remained *in utero*. The intrauterine levels are not necessarily relevant to the particular situation of the newborn VLBW infant and perhaps the best criteria we can obtain are the levels of *ad libitum* breast-fed full-term infants (8). Different groups of VLBW newborn infants have therefore been studied in order to provide a scale of comparison.

MATERIAL AND METHODS

The investigation was approved by the local Ethical Committee, and the parents gave their consent after having received verbal and written information. Twenty-five infants with birth weight below 1,800 g and gestational age below 34 weeks were divided into four groups (Table 1). The experimental period began as soon as the infants could tolerate 150 ml/kg per day intragastrically and ended at 36 weeks of postconceptional age. Heel-prick blood samples were obtained every second day during the first week and then weekly for the analysis of urea, calcium, sodium, potassium, base excess, and bicarbonate. An 8-hr urine collection was performed weekly for the analysis of sodium, potassium, calcium, and osmolality. Tyrosine was determined by a fluorimetric method, as this is a sensitive indicator of protein overload in the LBW newborn (9). Weight, length, and head circumference were plotted weekly on a perinatal growth curve (P. Karlberg, *personal communication*). All infants were without malformations and had an uncomplicated course during the observation period.

Whole-blood free amino acid levels were determined by a micro-method using capillary blood allowed to drop freely onto a filter paper. The equivalent of 10 μl of blood was eluted from the paper with physiological saline, deproteinized with sulfosalicylic acid, and freeze dried. The samples were stored at $-70°C$ before analysis on an automatic ion-exchange chromatography system (10). The reproducibility of the method was better than $\pm 5\%$ for the amino acids reported here.

TABLE 1. *The four feeding groups*

Parameter	Group A (n = 7)[a]		Group B (n = 6)[b]		Group C (n = 6)[c]		Group D (n = 6)[d]	
	Mean	Range	Mean	Range	Mean	Range	Mean	Range
Birth weight (g)	1,490	1,240–1,720	1,340	1,060–1,560	1,180	960–1,550	1,410	1,190–1,650
Gestation age (weeks)	30.6	29.0–32.0	30.2	28.0–32.0	28.0	27.0–32.0	30.8	28.0–34.0
Age when feeding regimen started (days)	11	10–16	15	10–21	22	12–35		

[a]Human milk protein (0.8 g) and human milk cream (1.0 g true fat) added to 100 ml of the mother's fresh milk (n = 5) or banked milk (n = 2) providing 125–140 kcal/kg per day and 3.0–3.4 g protein/kg per day.

[b]Human milk cream added to the mother's fresh milk (n = 3), to both mother's and banked milk, or to banked milk only (n = 1) providing 120–135 kcal/kg per day and 1.8–2.0 g protein/kg per day.

[c]Human milk protein added to mother's fresh milk (n = 3) or to banked milk (n = 3) providing 110–125 kcal/kg per day and 3.0–3.4 g protein/kg per day. Sodium chloride added giving a total amount of 20 mEq/liter.

[d]Mother's fresh milk only (n = 5) or both mother's milk and banked milk (n = 1) providing 105–120 kcal/kg per day and 1.8–2.0 g protein/kg per day.

Lactoengineering

The donors to the milk bank receive instructions for the hygienic collection of their milk and boil all contaminated parts of the electrical breast pump. Mothers are supplied with disinfected glass bottles into which the expressed breast milk is poured, cooled under running water, and then refrigerated. If the mother develops sore nipples, milk congestion, or infection, she is requested to call the milk bank. The donated milk is delivered to the local grocery store, where it is collected by the daily dairy products transportation. To be accepted for use, the bacterial concentration of the unpasteurized milk has to be below 100,000/ml. An acceptable milk is then pasteurized at 72°C for 15 sec (Alfa-Laval, type P 20-RB, modified plate heat exchanger).

Processing of the milk is shown in Fig. 2. The cream is separated in a simple Alfa-Laval separator type 100. The lactose and salts are separated by means of ultrafiltration through polysulfone membranes with a total area of 0.6 m² (the membrane from Kalle AG and the module from GKSS, West Germany). The milk is freeze dried in separate polypropylene cans (Hostalen PP, Hoechst) for 5 hr at − 20°C and for 48 hr at − 5°C (Hetosicc, CD 206, Hetolab Equipment AS, Denmark). Each can is cooled and stored under nitrogen. Bacterial controls are performed five times during the process.

The composition of the dry human milk powder is protein, 59.7%, fat, 7.7%, lactose, 10.9%, ash, 1.8%, Na, 0.12%, K, 0.24%, Ca, 0.49%, and Mg, 0.036%. In Group C, the supernatant of the "creamatocrit" (11) was used for sodium analysis, and sodium chloride was added to reach a final concentration of 20 mEq/liter, giving an osmolality of 320 mOsm/kg.

RESULTS

The growth rates of the infants in the different groups were similar. The group being given supplements of sodium chloride had similar serum sodium levels as the other groups (141 mM, range 131–148, $n = 6$; as against 139, range 134–145, $n = 17$), but higher concentrations of sodium in the urine (14 mM, range 4–25; as

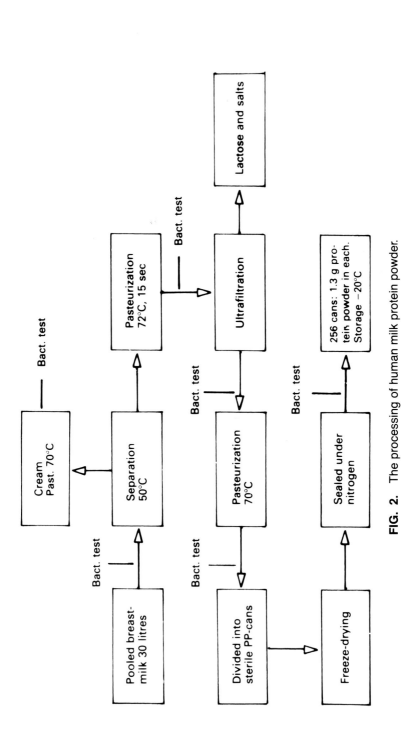

FIG. 2. The processing of human milk protein powder.

compared with 4, range 1–12). Serum urea was unaffected by the type of feeding, as were the other routine biochemical parameters (Table 2). The urinary C-peptide concentrations in the 6- to 8-hr urine were occasionally higher in the protein/calorie-imbalanced groups.

The whole-blood free amino acid levels for the "critical" amino acids indicating under- or overfeeding (5) are given in Fig. 3. The bars indicate the groups A, B, C, and D (from left to right). For comparison, the free amino acid levels of peripheral blood plasma of *ad libitum* breast-fed normal infants between 1 and 5 months of age (8) are indicated by a broken horizontal line. They correspond very closely with those of LBW infants given 170 ml/kg per day of pooled human milk determined by Rassin et al. (12,13).

It is evident from Fig. 3 that the blood amino acids show grossly elevated levels in the group supplemented with protein only (group C), whereas the addition of fat "normalized" the spectrum. The proline levels were elevated in group C, and low levels were seen in group B as compared to the unmodified human milk or the doubly supplemented group. In comparison to the plasma free amino acids of full-term breast-fed infants, the blood levels of the VLBW infants were generally lower except for tyrosine and glycine in the protein-only-supplemented group, where the levels were doubled. The plasma free amino acid levels of venous cord blood in term (14) and in premature deliveries (15) are generally higher (alanine and valine four times higher) than the blood levels of VLBW infants, again with the exception of glycine and tyrosine levels of the protein-only-substituted group, where the levels were twice as high.

DISCUSSION AND CONCLUSIONS

The absence of differences in growth rate between the infants who received protein-supplemented human milk and infants fed on preterm milk only has been demonstrated by others (7). Preterm milk has been reported to contain higher protein concentrations during the first weeks post-delivery (16); however, most of this increase is probably caused by secretory IgA (sIgA), which is not absorbed. In this study, the protein content was therefore assumed

TABLE 2. Results of the chemical analyses in the four groups after 2 weeks on the different feeding regimens (group D at 1 month of age)[a]

	Group A (n = 7)		Group B (n = 6)		Group C (n = 6)		Group D (n = 6)	
	Mean	Range	Mean	Range	Mean	Range	Mean	Range
Serum urea	4.3	1.7–7.6	2.5	1.7–3.2	4.1	2.9–5.6	4.1	1.6–8.3
Serum calcium	2.5	2.3–2.8	2.5	2.4–2.9	2.5	2.1–2.8	2.4	2.2–2.6
Blood base excess	+0.3	−4.0 to +3.1	−2.2	−3.8 to −1.0	−0.8	−4.2 to +1.8	−1.3	−5.0 to +3.3
Blood bicarbonate	23.5	21.0–26.7	23.4	21.2–27.9	23.2	20.7–24.3	24.4	22.0–26.7
Urinary calcium	2.0	1.2–3.0	3.5	1.0–6.4	5.3	1.5–16.8	2.0	0.6–3.9
Urinary mOsm/kg	100	70–165	113	90–155	162	80–315	87	55–160
Urinary C-peptide (nM)	1.7	1.0–2.6	2.9	1.1–6.1	2.8	1.1–9.5	1.2	0.3–2.5

[a]Urine collection is over 6–8 hr. Data expressed in millimoles unless otherwise indicated.

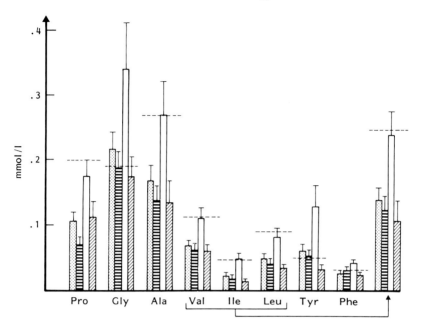

FIG. 3. Capillary whole blood free "critical" amino acid levels of 25 VLBW newborn infants (mean ± SE) in, from left to right, the four feeding groups A, B, C, and D. In group A the mother's milk was supplemented with human milk protein and fat, in group B with fat only, in group C with protein only, and in group D mother's own milk only was given. The differences between group C and the other groups are highly significant. The differences between the proline levels of groups A and B and the tyrosine levels of groups A and D are statistically significant ($p < 0.02$).

to be 1.2 g per 100 ml (based on N content), the addition providing a total of around 2 g per 100 ml of human formula. The total amount of sIgA (17) was 0.023 g/g of protein in the human milk protein isolate used. Moreover, the sIgA activity against a pool of eight *E. coli* O antigens, as measured by the ELISA method (18), was 57% of that of a reference milk pool. This may be potentially the most significant effect of raising the protein content of human milk for VLBW infants in this way, yielding a "hyperimmune breast milk."

The amino acid levels of plasma are lower than those of whole blood (19). Therefore, higher levels of free amino acids of blood plasma (full-term infants and cord blood) than those of whole blood (VLBW infants) cannot be explained by the fact that different amino acid pools were studied. "Normal" glycine levels (as compared to full-term breast-fed infants) and low alanine and branched-chain amino acid levels (valine, leucine, and isoleucine) of the doubly supplemented group, as well as the unfortified human-milk-fed group, at 150 to 175 ml/kg per day indicate (5) that the protein content of 3.0 to 3.4 g human milk protein/kg per day at a caloric intake of 125 to 140 kcal/kg per day is well tolerated. The imbalanced addition of protein only or fat only to the mother's milk produces an imbalance in the homeostasis of free amino acids in peripheral blood plasma. Since the brain uptake of free amino acids is correlated with the arterial levels (20), this could be disadvantageous to the supply of nutrients to the brain during this period of rapid brain growth.

Further investigations to reveal the optimal supply of protein will require the combination of the present methods with those of balance studies. A metabolic bed for incubators has been constructed, and such studies are in progress. An additional reason for adding human milk fat to the mother's own fresh milk is the presence of bile-salt-stimulated lipase activity in unprocessed human milk (21), which may contribute to the superior utilization of human milk lipids (22).

The human milk protein requirement will depend to some extent on the caloric intake achieved. The water and caloric requirements will depend on the external environment of the VLBW infants. The future development of firm recommendations on optimal protein intake will depend to a large extent on the more precise determination of optimal water and calorie requirements of the VLBW newborn infants during and after intensive neonatal care.

REFERENCES

1. Ziegler EE, Biga RL, Fomon SJ. In: Suskind RM, ed. Textbook of pediatric nutrition. New York: Raven Press, 1981:29–39.
2. Lindblad BS. In: Beard RW, Nathanielsz P, eds. Fetal physiology and medicine. Philadelphia: WB Saunders, 1976:80–104.
3. Lucas A, Lucas PJ, Chavin SI, Lyster RLJ, Baum JD. Early Hum Dev 1980;4(1):15–21.

4. Bell EF, Warburton D, Stuestreet BS, Oh W. N Engl J Med 1980;302:598–604.
5. Lindblad BS, Rahimtoola RJ, Hafiz-ur-Rehman R, et al. Acta Paediatr Scand 1978;67:335–43.
6. Hagelberg S, Lindblad BS, Lundsjö A, et al. Acta Paediatr Scand 1982;71:597–601.
7. Rönnholm KAR, Sipilä I, Siimes MA. J Pediatr 1982;101:243–7.
8. Lindblad BS, Alfvén G, Zetterström R. Acta Paediatr Scand 1978;67:659–63.
9. Waalkes TP, Udenfriend S. J Lab Clin Med 1959;50:733–6.
10. Spackman DH, Stein WH, Moore S. Anal Chem 1958;30:1190–205.
11. Lucas A, Gibbs JAH, Lyster RLJ, Baum JD. Br Med J 1978;1:1018–20.
12. Rassin DK, Gaull GE, Heinonen K, Räihä NCR. Pediatrics 1977;59:407–22.
13. Rassin DK, Gaull GE, Räihä NCR, Heinonen K. J Pediatr 1977;90:356–60.
14. Lindblad BS, Baldesten A. Acta Paediatr Scand 1967;56:37–48.
15. Lindblad BS, Zetterström R. Acta Paediatr Scand 1968;57:195–204.
16. Gross SJ, David RJ, Bauman L, Tomarelli RM. J Pediatr 1980;96:641–4.
17. Sohl Åkerlund A, Hanson LÅ, Alstedt S, Carlsson B. Scand J Immunol 1977;6:1275–82.
18. Ahlstedt S, Carlsson B, Hanson LÅ, Kaijser B, Mattsby Baltzer I, Sohl Åkerlund A. Scand J Immunol 1978;7:119–24.
19. Hagenfeldt L, Arvidsson A. Clin Chim Acta 1980;100:133–41.
20. Settergren G, Lindblad BS, Persson B. Acta Paediatr Scand 1976;65:343–53.
21. Fredrikzon B, Hernell O, Bläckberg L, Olivecrona T. Pediatr Res 1978;12:1048–52.
22. Alemi B, Hamosh M, Scanlon JW, Salzman-Mann C, Hamosh P. J Pediatr 1981;99:617–24.

Human Milk Banking, edited by
A. F. Williams and J. D. Baum.
Nestlé Nutrition, Vevey/Raven Press,
New York © 1984.

Nitrogen, Fat, and Mineral Balance Studies in Low-Birth-Weight Infants Fed with Banked Human Milk, Human Milk Formula, or Preterm Infant Formula

*Jacques Senterre, **Marcel Voyer, †Guy Putet, and
*Jacques Rigo

*Department of Neonatal Pediatrics, State University of Liège, Hôpital de
Bavière, 4020 Liège, Belgium; **Institut de Puériculture de Paris,
Paris, France; and †University Hospital Edouard Herriot, Lyons, France

The best food for low-birth-weight (LBW) infants remains controversial. Because of its immunological properties and nutritional qualities, human milk is considered the superior food for all neonates. It has been shown that preterm infants may benefit from their own mother's milk made richer in protein and electrolytes than mature breast milk (1). However, following premature delivery, breast milk is not always available.

Because of its low protein, energy, and mineral content, banked human milk is often considered inadequate to fulfill the nutritional requirements of rapidly growing LBW infants (2,3). On the other hand, feeding with standard formulas often leads to a high fecal loss of fat, which decreases the amount of energy available for growth and impedes calcium absorption and nitrogen retention (4–6). Therefore, in recent years, human milk lactoengineering and specially adapted formulas have been developed to meet the specific nutritional needs of LBW infants.

The aim of the present chapter is to compare the results of metabolic balances carried out in three groups of very LBW infants

171

fed either banked human milk, human milk formula, or LBW infant formula.

MATERIALS AND METHODS

Thirty 3-day metabolic balance studies were carried out in three groups of matched healthy male preterm infants fed either pasteurized banked human milk, human milk formula, or LBW infant formula. Mean gestational age was 30 ± 2 weeks, and mean birth weight $1,280 \pm 190$ g. Each infant was given only one type of milk from the age of 10 days, when intake volume reached ~ 180 ml/kg per day. Daily vitamin D intake was 30 μg (1,200 I.U.) from birth (6). Metabolic balances were carried out at 27 ± 7 days of age.

The human milk formula was made by adding to 1 liter of partially skimmed human milk (fat content: 1.2 ± 0.9 g) 35 g of lyophilized whole human milk, 12 g of medium-chain triglycerides (MCT), 6 g of linoleate, and 92 mg of phosphorus ($K_2H\ PO_4$). Mean compositions of banked human milk, human milk formula, and LBW infant formula are given in Table 1. The balance studies were performed in a hammock-shaped metabolic bed inside an incubator, as previously described (7). Total nitrogen, fat, and minerals were measured in milk, homogenized stools, and urine

TABLE 1. *Mean composition of banked human milk (HM), human milk formula (HMF) and low-birth-weight infant formula (LBWIF)*

Amount per 100 ml	HM	HMF	LBWIF
Total nitrogen (mg)	215	301	302
Total fat (g)	2.9	3.8	3.3
MCT (%)	—	30	40
Lactose (g)	6.4	7.4	7.2
Dextrins (g)	—	—	2.4
Calcium (mg)	29	36	57
Magnesium (mg)	3.0	3.1	4.5
Phosphorus (mg)	13	21	39
Energy (kcal)	57	71	76

using respectively a micro-Kjeldahl technique, a gravimetric method, and atomic absorption spectroscopy.

All results were expressed as means ± 1 SD, and statistical analysis was carried out using Student's *t*-test.

RESULTS

Mean daily weight gain per kilogram body weight from the day the child reached its birth weight again was 13.5 g with banked human milk, 17.4 g with human milk formula, and 20.9 g with LBW infant formula. The metabolic balance data are presented in Table 2.

Net protein intakes (N × 6.25) were higher (3.4 versus 2.5 g/kg/ day) in the infants fed human milk formula or LBW infant formula than in those fed banked human milk. Net absorption of nitrogen was significantly higher (88% versus 81%) in the infants fed the cow's-milk-based formula than in those fed human milk. Urinary excretion of nitrogen was lowest with banked human milk (81 mg/ kg/day). It increased by about 50% with the human milk formula or the LBW infant formula. Nevertheless, mean nitrogen retention was significantly higher in the infants fed the human milk formula (317 mg/kg/day) or the LBW infant formula (356 mg/kg/day) than in those fed banked human milk (242 mg/kg/day).

The coefficients of fat absorption were lower in the infants fed banked human milk (69 ± 11%) or the human milk formula (76 ± 12%) than in those fed the LBW infant formula (87 ± 6%).

Intake and fecal loss of calcium were about twice as high in the infants fed the LBW infant formula than in those fed banked human milk or human milk formula. Net absorption of calcium was slightly but not significantly higher (70% versus 60%) in the human-milk-fed infants than in those artificially fed. Calcium retention was 64 mg/kg/day with the LBW infant formula, 38 mg/kg/day with the human milk formula, and 23 mg/kg/day with banked human milk.

Phosphorus intake was about twice as high in the artificially fed infants than in those fed human milk. However, because of phosphorus supplementation, phosphorus intake was slightly higher in

TABLE 2. *Results (mean ± 1 SD) of metabolic balance studies in very-low-birth-weight infants fed either banked human milk (HM), a human milk formula (HMF), or a low-birth-weight infant formula (LBWIF)*

Intake or output (mg/kg/day)	HM (n = 10)	HMF (n = 10)	LBWIF (n = 10)
Nitrogen			
Intake	398 ± 28	553 ± 43	542 ± 33
Feces	75 ± 15	105 ± 17	67 ± 20
Urine	81 ± 17	132 ± 26	119 ± 30
Retention	242 ± 31	317 ± 42	356 ± 30
Fat			
Intake (g)	5.8 ± 0.9	7.0 ± 2.1	6.0 ± 0.3
Feces (g)	1.8 ± 0.6	1.7 ± 1.0	0.8 ± 0.3
Absorption (%)	69 ± 11	76 ± 12	87 ± 6
Calcium			
Intake	55 ± 9	63 ± 7	111 ± 7
Feces	18 ± 9	19 ± 10	45 ± 16
Urine	14 ± 6	6 ± 4	2 ± 1
Retention	23 ± 10	38 ± 13	64 ± 14
Phosphorus			
Intake	25 ± 4	36 ± 5	71 ± 8
Feces	3 ± 1	3 ± 1	6 ± 3
Urine	Traces	1 ± 1	17 ± 2
Retention	22 ± 5	32 ± 4	48 ± 7
Magnesium			
Intake	5.7 ± 0.3	5.8 ± 0.4	7.6 ± 0.5
Feces	2.9 ± 1.0	3.0 ± 1.1	4.6 ± 1.3
Urine	1.1 ± 0.4	0.9 ± 0.3	0.6 ± 0.4
Retention	1.7 ± 1.1	1.9 ± 1.0	2.4 ± 1.7

the infants fed the human formula than in those fed banked human milk. Net absorption of phosphorus was about 90% in the three groups. Urinary excretion of phosphorus was practically zero in the two groups fed human milk, whereas it reached 17 mg/kg/day in the group fed the LBW infant formula. Nevertheless, phosphorus retention was highest in the latter group.

Magnesium intakes averaged 5.7 mg/kg/day in the two groups fed human milk and 7.6 mg/kg/day in the group artificially fed.

Magnesium absorption tended to be higher in the infants fed human milk, but urinary excretion of magnesium was also higher. Magnesium retention represented about one-third of the intake in the three groups.

DISCUSSION

In nutritional guidelines for the feeding of preterm infants, reference is often made to the growth rate and the accumulation of nutrients *in utero* (3). In the present study, the weight gain of infants fed human milk formula was similar to that achieved *in utero*. It was lower for the infants fed banked human milk and higher for those fed the LBW infant formula.

The fetal accumulation rate of nitrogen is ~340 mg/kg/day between 30 and 36 weeks of gestation, i.e., ~2% of the weight gain (8). Similar retention of nitrogen was observed in the infants fed the human milk formula or the LBW infant formula, whereas it was about two-thirds of this value in infants fed banked human milk. However, in the three groups, nitrogen retention represented about 2% of the weight gain.

The relatively high fecal loss of nitrogen in the infants fed human milk has already been reported (4). It might be attributable to the acceleration of the transit time and the presence of poorly degraded immunoglobulins. The low nitrogen retention in the group of infants fed banked human milk can be explained by the low nitrogen intake. Indeed, low urinary excretion of nitrogen shows that the amount of nitrogen absorbed is utilized mainly for protein synthesis. Although the nitrogen intakes were higher in the infants fed the human milk formula and the LBW infant formula, urinary excretion of nitrogen was only slightly increased in those two groups. The good utilization of the protein intake in this case is probably related to the higher caloric intake and the better absorption of fat (4).

Poor absorption of fat in LBW infants fed heat-treated human milk has been already observed (9) and is probably related to the inactivation of the bile-salt-stimulated lipase (10). The better fat absorption observed in the infants fed the human milk formula or the LBW infant formula can be explained by the presence of well-absorbed medium-chain triglycerides, which constitute 30 to 40% of the total fat (11).

A number of factors such as calcium–phosphorus ratio in the milk, fecal loss of fat, intestinal secretion of endogenous calcium, intake and metabolism of vitamin D, and postnatal age have all been implicated in calcium absorption by LBW infants (6). In previous studies, we have shown that vitamin D is hydroxylated in the liver and the kidney (12,13) and that 1,25-dihydroxyvitamin D is the major factor regulating intestinal absorption of calcium in the premature infant (14). High vitamin D intake certainly accounted for the good calcium absorption observed in the present study (6). The poor calcium retention in the infants fed banked human milk can be explained by the low calcium intake and the high urinary excretion of calcium. Hypercalciuria is caused by the relative lack of phosphorus; it can be corrected by supplementing milk with phosphate, as has been demonstrated previously (15). The higher urinary excretion of magnesium in the group fed banked human milk is probably also a result of low phosphorus intake.

In conclusion, feeding human milk to preterm infants has the advantage of providing antiinfectious factors, excluding foreign proteins, and minimizing metabolic stress. However, as shown in the present study, pasteurized banked human milk is not fully adequate for feeding very LBW infants. The caloric density is rather low, and the fat is poorly absorbed. Nitrogen retention reaches only two-thirds of the nitrogen accumulation rate *in utero* because of the milk's low nitrogen content. In addition, its low mineral content, especially of phosphorus, is frequently responsible for bone hypomineralization. In view of the uniqueness of human milk, a human milk formula richer in energy, nitrogen, and minerals, including phosphorus, appears to be more suitable for feeding very LBW infants when the mother's milk is not available. However human milk lactoengineering is expensive and time consuming. When human milk is not available, feeding a specially adapted formula such as the one used in the present study may be an acceptable alternative from the nutritional point of view.

REFERENCES

1. Gross SJ, David RJ, Baumna L, Tomarelli RM. J Pediatr 1980;96:641–4.
2. Atkinson SA, Anderson GH, Bryan MH. Am J Clin Nutr 1980;33:811–5.
3. Ziegler EE, Biga RL, Fomon SJ. In: Suskind RM, ed. Pediatric nutrition. New York: Raven Press, 1979:29–39.
4. Senterre J. In: Visser HKA, ed. Nutrition and metabolism of the fetus and infant. The Hague: Martinus Nijhoff, 1979:195–212.
5. Senterre J. In: Arneil GC, Metcoff J, eds. BIMR-Pediatrics Vol. 3 Nutrition 1984 Chap 5 1–12. London: Butterworths (in press).
6. Senterre J, Salle B. Acta Paediatr Scand 1982; Suppl. 296:85–92.
7. Senterre J, Sodoyez-Goffaux F, Lambrechts A. Acta Paediatr Belg 1971;25:133–42.
8. Shaw JCL. Pediatr Clin North Am 1973;20:333–58.
9. Williamson S, Finucane E, Ellis H, Gamsu HR. Arch Dis Child 1978;53:555–63.
10. Hernell O, Bläckberg L, Fredrikzon B, Olivecrona T. In: Lebenthal E, ed. Textbook of gastroenterology and nutrition in infancy. New York: Raven Press, 1981:465–71.
11. Roy CC, Ste-Marie M, Chartrand L, Weber A, Bard H, Doray B. J Pediatr 1975;86:446–50.
12. Glorieux FH, Salle B, Delvin CE, David L. J Pediatr 1981;99:640–3.
13. Salle B, Glorieux FH, Delvin EE, David LS, Meunier G. Acta Paediatr Scand 1983;72:203–6.
14. Senterre J, David L, Salle B. In: Stern L, Salle B, Friis-Hansen B., eds. Intensive care in the newborn, vol. III. New York: Masson, 1981:115–25.
15. Senterre J, Putet G, Salle B, Rigo J. J Pediatr (in press).

Human Milk Banking, edited by
A. F. Williams and J. D. Baum.
Nestlé Nutrition, Vevey/Raven Press,
New York © 1984.

Human Milk Processing and the Nutrition of the Very-Low-Birth-Weight Infant: Discussion

A. F. Williams and J. D. Baum

*University Department of Paediatrics, John Radcliffe Hospital,
Oxford OX3 9DU, England*

A principal effect of juxtaposing presentations of *in vitro* biochemical experiments and clinical studies was disclosure of the gap between *in vitro* observation and the demonstration of a clinical effect. It is easy to argue teleologically that because a substance is present in milk it has a function; however, in most cases we have little clinical evidence that this is the case. The discussion was therefore devoted to the formulation of clinical questions about the use of human milk for feeding low-birth-weight infants and to suggestions as to how the investigation of these questions might be approached.

Dr. W. A. Silverman prefaced the discussion by outlining how much neonatal feeding regimens had changed over his 40 years of clinical practice, pointing out the need for clinical trials "to challenge by design and scepticism when confronted with making the enormous step from observation to clinical practice." He outlined the need to begin with an exact question and reiterated the serious problems of subject heterogeneity and therapeutic cointerventions in conducting such trials. Distinguishing between pragmatic and explanatory clinical trials, he made the point that cointervention is less of a problem in the former. Pragmatic trials merely compare treatments between equivalent and concurrently treated groups and are preferably collaborative, since this increases the legitimacy of generalizing from their conclusions to make operational decisions about clinical practice. In the case of the explanatory trial, in which a more direct link between cause and effect is sought, the need to standardize the conditions other than the one being studied often makes it difficult to generalize results because of the artificiality of the trial conditions. A further point was the requirement for a prestudy prediction of the difference in outcome measure expected. This is, in itself, a difficult estimate to make without a clear appreciation of the basic patterns of early postnatal growth in very-low-birth-weight (VLBW) infants.

From these generalizations, the discussion moved to consideration of separate questions that were relevant to the subject. These were threefold:

1. Should human milk be pasteurized before it is given to VLBW babies?
2. How might the effects of feeding supplemented human milk to VLBW babies be measured?
3. By what objective tests can the physiological functions of individual milk constituents, such as secretory IgA and growth factors, be shown to be of importance to human infants?

These questions were discussed separately to illustrate some of the problems of designing clinical trials given the limited power of the experimental methods commonly employed.

SHOULD HUMAN MILK BE PASTEURIZED BEFORE IT IS GIVEN TO VLBW BABIES?

Apart from a few isolated case reports, there is little evidence to incriminate donor human milk as a vector of nosocomial infection in newborn nurseries. Indeed, in southern Sweden unpasteurized human milk has been given to babies for many years. Nevertheless, caution needs to be exercised in generalizing that because unpasteurized human milk is safely given in Sweden, the practice would be safe in all parts of the world and in all societies. On the other hand, there is some *in vitro* evidence that heat treatment may be deleterious to milk constituents. However, a problem in assessing the significance of *in vitro* studies is that time–temperature cycles used for batch pasteurization have, in most cases, not been accurately reproduced in the laboratory. This is an important consideration, since the effects of heating are critically dependent on the time–temperature cycle that is employed. From the point of view of current clinical practice, therefore, the decision as to whether milk is to be pasteurized or not is largely one of personal opinion based on the above considerations. What is needed is a comparative clinical study between equivalent and concurrently treated groups of infants fed either pasteurized or unpasteurized donor human milk.

Two clinical questions require answering. First, does heat treatment affect nutrient absorption from donor human milk? Second, does heat treatment reduce the antimicrobial protection that we assume the infant receives from donor human milk?

The first question is of a different order from the second and could probably be answered by balance studies in small groups of infants in a single nursery, in other words, by an explanatory clinical trial. The second question is more complex because of the low incidence of proven infection in neonatal nurseries in Western countries. It would obviously require a large collaborative study for any difference in infection rates to become apparent. Furthermore, if the overall incidence of proven infection among VLBW infants receiving donor human milk is below 15%, what would we take as a substantial difference in infection rate in making the prestudy prediction? Furthermore, a sufficiently large trial in the Western countries would clearly introduce many organizational problems. For example, how would milk composition be standardized? And how would observer blindness be ensured? The latter would clearly be of great importance because of the possible bias that might be introduced if the observer had a different threshold to investigate and treat presumed infected episodes in the group receiving unpasteurized milk. Conceivably, the size of the trial could be reduced by conducting the trial in a nursery situated in a less developed country, where infection accounts for a much greater part of morbidity amongst VLBW infants.

HOW MIGHT THE EFFECTS OF
FEEDING SUPPLEMENTED HUMAN MILK TO
VLBW INFANTS BE MEASURED?

Again, small explanatory trials might answer some of the questions about the short-term effects of nutritional supplementation on infants' growth. However, it seems likely that, given small numbers, an effect would only be demonstrated in well infants. The reason for this is difficulty in standardizing and controlling cointerventions when studying sick VLBW infants. Such trials must also be interpreted with caution, as errors could be made in generalizing from their conclusions. Would one be justified, for instance, in extrapolating findings from well VLBW infants to sick VLBW infants? Ironically, it is studies on sick VLBW infants that are most urgently required, since, theoretically, malnutrition may compound the effects of other perinatal insults. How might such effects be measured in the long term? Professor J. Dobbing pointed out the difficulty of separating developmental effects attributable to minor differences in nutritional intake from those attributable to other environmental influences on VLBW infants. In other words, very large trials (i.e., with sufficient statistical power) might be carried out and no difference observed be attributable to problems of nutrition not because there were no such effects but because the clinical instruments were too coarse for their detection.

BY WHAT OBJECTIVE TESTS CAN
THE PHYSIOLOGICAL FUNCTIONS OF INDIVIDUAL
MILK CONSTITUENTS BE SHOWN TO BE OF
IMPORTANCE TO HUMAN INFANTS?

This discussion was centered on secretory immunoglobulin A as a specific milk component. Current knowledge of human milk secretory immunoglobulin A synthesis and its response to oral immunization of the mother strongly suggests that secretory immunoglobulin A has a role in passive protection of the neonatal gut. What is now needed is objective evidence of clinical advantage from such immunoglobulin A for the VLBW infant.

The prophylactic role of secretory immunoglobulin A in protecting infants from infection would require the study of either a large number of infants in developed countries or smaller numbers of infants in the less-developed countries. However, human milk resources might prove insufficient to provide the quantities of human secretory immunoglobulin A required for such a trial. As an alternative, one might be able to demonstrate an effect of supplementary secretory immunoglobulin A in a specific condition such as infantile gastroenteritis. More exploratory work is needed before a clinical trial could be mounted in order to establish what the necessary origin (and hence the bacterial specificity) of the immunoglobulin A should be and what minimum dose would be required to demonstrate an effect. Since supplies of human milk proteins are likely to be a limiting factor in mounting such trials, perhaps the effects of antimicrobial mediators from milks of other species (e.g., bovine lactoperoxidase and immunoglobulins) might be considered worthy of therapeutic trial.

Our limited understanding of the physicochemical nature of other factors in human milk, e.g., some of the growth modulators referred to by Dr. Gaull and co-workers *(this volume)*, is at present an obstacle to framing the appropriate precise question that would be required before a clinical trial could be contemplated.

These questions illustrate the complexity of the problems involved in studying the nutrition of VLBW infants. It is clear that narrowing the area of uncertainty in each case will not be easy.

Subject Index